LIVING WITH PROSTATE CANCER

LIVING WITH PROSTATE CANCER

One Man's Story

———— • ————

What Everyone Should Know

Audrey Currie Newton

M&S

Canadian Cataloguing in Publication Data

Newton, Audrey Currie, date
   Living with prostate cancer: one man's story: what everyone should know

Includes bibliographical references and index.
ISBN 0-7710-6779-8

1. Newton, Victor, d. 1991 – Health. 2. Prostate – Cancer – Patients – Biography.
I. Title.

RC280.P7N49 1996   362.1'9699463'0092   C95-933377-0

The publisher acknowledges the support of the Canada Council and the Ontario Arts Council for their publishing program.

Illustrations: John McLachlan
Typesetting: M&S, Toronto
Printed and bound in Canada on acid-free paper

McClelland & Stewart Inc.
The Canadian Publishers
481 University Avenue
Toronto, Ontario
M5G 2E9

1 2 3 4 5   00 99 98 97 96

• CONTENTS •

Audrey Newton has written a moving account of her husband's long and, at times, desperate battle with prostate cancer. Approximately 14,000 new cases of this disease are diagnosed in Canada annually, so Audrey's story is being repeated, with different twists and turns in every case, again and again, hundreds and perhaps thousands of times. Certainly it is not unusual to read that the diagnosis was late, nor that despite the advanced nature of the disease at discovery, her husband lived another ten years and more.

Personal encounters with prostate cancer have provided material for a number of publications. Cornelius Ryan, more famous for his books *A Bridge Too Far* and *The Longest Day*, told his story about a losing battle with prostate cancer in a book entitled *A Private Battle*. Tom Alexander wrote a lengthy article in *Fortune* magazine (September 20, 1993) about his own prostate cancer. What struck me about both accounts, and Audrey's as well, was how angry all three writers were, at times, at particular members of the medical profession and, at the same time, how laudatory they were of others. As a worker in the field, I found it both puzzling and frustrating that neither the anger nor the praise appeared to be related to the quality of the advice or service rendered. Often, I got the impression plaudits correlated with how closely the advice approximated the writer's own point of view – right or wrong.

Alexander's article, for example, chastises doctors who will not consider treatment options other than surgery for his disease. He then elects to be looked after by a young doctor who agrees with him to simply follow the progress of his disease. This particular doctor is praised to the hilt. Meanwhile, Alexander's PSA is rising and, in my opinion, he may be missing the "window of opportunity" to obtain a cure. Ryan, I recall, vented his anger at the chief of a famous cancer institute whose advice, in my reading, was perfectly sound. Audrey Newton, in this book, applauds the doctors at the Princess Margaret Hospital at the expense of the Toronto General. But, in my view, the Toronto General treated her husband appropriately, as far as the science was concerned. What all this suggests to me is that communication skills and compassion are as important as surgical skills and science when we are dealing with cancer. Doctors who lose sight of this fact or choose to ignore it will have angry and hostile patients fleeing their care no matter how correct their ministration.

I hope this book finds a wide audience. The claim has been made, and widely circulated in the media, that nothing can or should be done when prostate cancer is discovered. We need to refute this. Would Audrey's husband have lived as long without the radiotherapy or the hormonal therapy? I doubt it. Epidemiologists quote figures to show that patients live just as long with and without treatment. These survival figures, however, reflect neither the impact of PSA blood testing, nor that of ultrasound-guided needle biopsy, both measures which have made earlier diagnosis more likely than it was even a decade ago.

Prostate cancer is a curable cancer made incurable by a delayed diagnosis. Audrey Newton's warm and accurate account of the ravages of prostate cancer may prompt other men to seek earlier attention for symptoms that point to prostate gland disease. That would be justification enough for her effort. If, however, men and the medical profession choose to ignore early diagnosis and treatment as worthwhile options, we will be allowing this cancer to overtake lung cancer to become the number one cancer killer of men.

Yosh Taguchi, M.D., Ph.D., F.R.C.S.C., Program Director of Urology, McGill University, and Senior Urologist, Royal Victoria Hospital, Montreal, is the author of *Private Parts: An Owner's Guide*.

For Victor, a promise kept

I remember clearly the day Victor received the results of his first biopsy. He said he felt as though the world were standing still. The doctor was speaking but Victor didn't hear a word he said. As Victor recalled later, when he heard the word "cancer," he was filled with the fear of death. I remember that I, too, was confused when I heard the news, my mind crowded with a thousand questions. When we emerged from the doctor's office, only one thing was clear and certain: we had entered another world, the world of cancer and all it contained.

This is the story of how Victor and I learned about and coped with his prostate cancer. Cancer, we discovered, is not only a matter of visits to doctors and hospitals and accepting treatment. It is a disease that brings with it radical and irreversible change. It is an enemy whose presence engaged us in a constant battle. It invaded every aspect of our daily lives – our working, eating, and sleeping habits, our sex lives, and our relationships with family and friends.

We fought it with all the resources we could draw on. We found strength within ourselves greater than we knew we had.

We depended upon each other perhaps more than ever before. And we armed ourselves with information. There are some people, I realize, who prefer not to know everything about their illness. They would prefer to put themselves in the hands of medical professionals and hope for the best. This was not our way. There are many reliable (and some not so reliable) sources of knowledge about cancer and its treatment. We sought out books and articles on the subject and asked our doctors to explain everything. We found that the knowledge we acquired helped prepare us for the trials that Victor had to endure and that it dispelled at least some of our fears and misapprehensions. I would urge any couple who find themselves in a similar situation to do as we did and learn all they can about their own particular cancer.

Victor and I fought the battle together. The fact that he had cancer in no way diminished our feeling for each other. Our lives were changed, of course, but it was not all for the worse. We met others along the way who were less lucky than we were. We saw marriages that were not able to withstand cancer's assault and individuals, left to fend for themselves, who gave up the struggle at an early stage. There's no question that the victim of prostate cancer needs the practical help and emotional support of another person, whether a spouse, lover, family member, or close friend.

I wrote this book for two reasons. First, I wanted men and women to learn about the prostate gland and the diseases – especially cancer – that can affect it. Secondly, I wanted to convey some sense of the tremendous emotional impact this disease can have upon those who are afflicted by it so that the reader will have a better understanding of what they may have to contend with.

The book is divided into four parts, each of which corre-—
sponds roughly with a distinct stage in the course of the disease.
The first part deals with the initial symptoms and diagnosis; the
second with the treatments and procedures that may be applied
in particular cases; the third with the everyday problems
patients and caregivers may encounter when they live with the
disease; the fourth, finally, deals with the last stages of the
disease, when palliative care takes the place of attempts either
to reverse or stop its progress.

Each part, in turn, has two sections. In the brief opening sections, I have attempted to explain the plain facts: what you
should know about prostate cancer. Then, in the succeeding
pages, I have told the story of Victor's struggle with the disease.
Readers will also find a list of information, including books and
organizations, at the end of the book.

Many threads run through all cancer stories. By describing
what Victor went through, I have tried to emphasize those
aspects of his experience that all, or many, patients have in
common. I hope that this book will serve others as a reliable
guide. But, for all that they may share, everyone who contracts
prostate cancer also has his own unique experience. Every
patient, and the people who care for and support him, should
also look for information from other sources. This book is
meant to be a reliable general reference. It is definitely not a
substitute for the advice of a qualified physician.

As a courtesy, and as a matter of discretion, I have disguised
the identity of some individuals in telling this story.

An effort has been made in these pages to provide the reader with basic information about the medical diagnosis and treatment of prostate cancer. This information is of a general nature only. It is not a substitute for a physician's advice. Doctors disagree among themselves about the effectiveness of some diagnostic tools and medical therapies. In addition, the results of ongoing research may lead to the reassessment of established routines and to the adoption of new therapies. No attempt has been made in this book to explore or resolve the issues over which doctors disagree or to anticipate new directions in treatment. For further guidance in a particular case readers are urged to seek the assistance of a qualified medical doctor.

Symptoms and Diagnosis

Most men know very little about the prostate gland. They may know only that it has something to do with sex and that it is "down there" somewhere. Of course, as long as the gland is healthy and functioning normally, there is no reason to learn more. Only when symptoms develop does the spirit of enquiry begin to flourish.

The Anatomy of the Prostate Gland

The prostate gland sits just beneath the bladder in front of the rectum (Figure 1). It's about the size of a walnut or golf ball. By inserting a gloved finger into the rectum, a doctor can easily feel the prostate gland through the wall of the lower bowel. The urethra, the tube that carries urine from the bladder to the outside, runs through the prostate.

When the prostate is diseased, it often swells, reducing or cutting off the flow of urine (Figure 2). If you can imagine a ring around the middle of a garden hose becoming tighter and tighter, cutting off the flow of water, then you have an idea of how a troubled prostate can interfere with the ability to urinate.

What Does It Do?

The prostate gland manufactures part of the fluid that makes semen. Semen is the whitish fluid that carries the sperm produced by the testicles, the same fluid that is discharged when a man ejaculates. In order to make semen, the prostate needs testosterone, a hormone that is also produced largely by the testicles. Testosterone plays a significant part in the reproductive cycle. It is the male sex hormone responsible for the development of male sexual characteristics. It also promotes the growth of both benign and malignant prostatic tissue.

Symptoms to Watch For

Many men ignore the first symptoms that indicate prostate trouble. Don't! Virtually all problems can be treated, and some can be cured, but it is always better to catch these troubles sooner rather than later. Here are the symptoms you should acknowledge and be aware of. Call your doctor and make an appointment now, if you have one or more of these symptoms:

- the urge to urinate frequently, especially at night
- difficulty getting your stream started
- a stream that starts and stops
- a burning sensation when you urinate
- painful ejaculation
- blood in your semen or urine
- pain in your lower spine or between the scrotum and anus
- an unusually bloated abdomen.

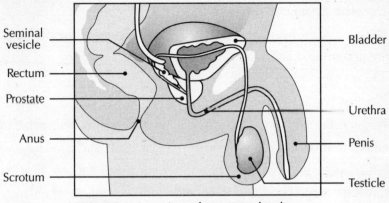

FIGURE 1: Location of prostate gland.

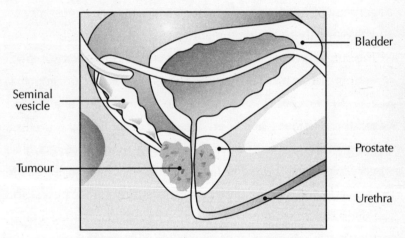

FIGURE 2: Prostate cancer: tumour puts
pressure on urethra, interfering with flow
of urine from bladder.

Any or all of these symptoms can signal a problem. Prostate
problems occur in 50 per cent of men age sixty and over. Only a
medical doctor can accurately determine what kind of problem
an individual is having and how best to treat it.

The Most Common Problems

The symptoms listed above may indicate the presence of one of the following diseases or conditions.

Benign Prostatic Hyperplasia (or Hypertrophy) (BPH)
This condition is simply an enlarged prostate gland. About half of all North American men over fifty have an enlarged prostate and it is proportionately more common in men over the age of sixty. It is a treatable condition. Depending on the degree of enlargement, either drugs (usually in the early stage) or surgery (in the later stage) may be recommended. The treatments are almost always effective and there is little threat to sexual function.

The surgical procedure for treating BPH is called transurethral resection of the prostate (TURP) and is performed on approximately 20 per cent of men who have enlarged prostate glands. When the prostate gland is enlarged, it compresses the urethra, causing problems with urination among many sufferers. The surgery to remedy these problems is performed by a urologist. He pushes a device into the urethra, entering through the penis, and removes the innermost core of the enlarged prostate gland, leaving the tough outer layer intact and relieving the pressure on the urethra. The operation lasts about one or two hours and entails a short hospital stay of a few days to a week, depending on the patient's state of health.

Most men worry about the effect on their sex life of this kind of operation. The ability to get an erection does not usually change; however, a small percentage of men do experience some postoperative sexual difficulties.

Because only part of the prostate gland is removed in this

procedure, it is still possible to develop prostate cancer and all men, whether or not they have been diagnosed with enlarged prostates, should continue to have annual examinations of their prostates.

Prostatitis

Prostatitis is an inflammation or infection of the prostate gland. It is usually treated with anti-inflammatory agents and antibiotics. Again, there is almost no threat to sexual function.

Cancer of the Prostate Gland

Cancer of the prostate begins with an abnormal growth of cells that divide and multiply over a period of years, eventually producing a lump or nodule. At some point, the growth is likely to put pressure on the urethra or otherwise cause the patient discomfort or pain. At this stage it may be detected either by a doctor conducting a rectal examination or by a transrectal ultrasound test. The abnormal growth is called a tumour. Not all tumours are cancerous. Some are benign (non-cancerous) and do not spread (metastasize) to other parts of the body. The malignant cells that form cancerous tumours are dangerous because they never stop multiplying. They take up space and rob healthy cells of nourishment. Eventually, they find their way into the lymphatic system or blood stream where they can spread to any part of the body.

Victor was getting up at night more and more often. I couldn't help noticing it and I mentioned it to him several times. He insisted that he was fine. He said that he had always gotten up a few times at night. When I told him he should see a doctor he just got angry.

I was becoming concerned and I knew that it was bothering him more than he would admit. One morning I tried to force the issue. Still he refused to talk to me about it. He just gulped his coffee and walked past me. "I'll be in the woods if you need me," he said, and slammed the door shut behind him.

Once he was outside he called to Cleo, our big Newfoundland dog. "C'mon girl, let's see if we can clear some of the bush on the back forty." The "back forty" was something of an exaggeration. We had about ten acres of land behind the old stone schoolhouse near the town of Warkworth, Ontario, where we had moved six years ago, a few months before we were married in 1975. I was then thirty-nine and Victor was fifty-three.

Victor loved the woods and the old schoolhouse. He had put an immense amount of work into the property. He had converted the house itself into a country home with beautifully landscaped lawns and lush gardens. He had made an art studio out of an old storage shed at the back of the house. A true labour of love, the studio became a love nest and refuge whenever we wanted a change of scene. It wasn't without reason that he installed a potbellied stove, built a sofa bed into one wall, and cut a large picture window overlooking the property into another. Viewed from that window, the fruit and lilac trees seemed to be in constant motion, inhabited in all seasons by a variety of birds.

It was not to the studio that Victor headed when he wanted to avoid talking to me, however, but to the bush behind it. There, with Cleo beside him, he sat down on a log and reached for a cigarette. The gesture was unconscious, a matter of habit: the cigarettes were no longer there. He had given up smoking a year before, along with the five Scotches he used to drink before dinner.

His quitting drinking was the result of a series of arguments over a long period. Although he had never been abusive when he drank, his demeanour changed under the influence, and I told him so. I had packed my bags more than once and fled to Toronto for a few days of solace with my brother Joe. Victor always called and apologized. And then he would meet me with flowers and kisses at the train station when I came back. And then the sequence would be repeated.

Finally, I had given him an ultimatum: either he would give up hard liquor or I would not return. He wrote me a letter when I had been gone for a week and in it he said a lot of tears had been shed as he walked the country road alone. I returned and he never drank liquor again, taking only one glass of wine with his dinner. Years later when he was asked how he could give it up, he answered, "It was easy. I happen to love my wife."

Now, sitting on a log with Cleo as his companion, he looked with a glum countenance at the house. He hated arguing with me. He knew he would not be clearing brush from the path at the back of the house, or setting his mind to do anything else, until he made up with me. "Come on, Cleo," he said finally, and rubbed the big dog's head. "Let's find Audrey."

"Who loves who around here anyway?" He handed me the last of the autumn flowers from the garden. I moved quickly to his open arms.

"Let's see. I love you," I said, "and you love Cleo and Cleo loves me and everybody loves everybody around here."

~

A week later I brought the subject up again. "Victor dear," I said softly, choosing an occasion when he was feeling mellow, "you are going to turn sixty soon."

"That's right," he agreed, "January 2nd, 1982."

"What I'm suggesting, sweetheart, is that you really should think about having a check-up. I know you're fine, but men your age should have their hearts checked, just to be on the safe side." I snuggled against his broad chest and listened to the strong, regular beat of his heart. Of course, it wasn't his heart that worried me; it was his frequent trips to the bathroom and his unspoken yet obvious distress.

I had studied medical texts on my own for most of my adult years. I knew that Victor had a problem with his urinary tract and that it was becoming progressively worse. I knew he would eventually have to seek a doctor's help, but if a malignancy were found, something I had not discounted for a minute, then any delay in getting treatment was dangerous.

I had grown up with an awareness of cancer. My brother Gerald died of leukaemia when he was eleven. Hardly anyone knew what leukaemia was in those days, so my mother simply called it "cancer," and everyone understood.

There was no way of telling what the root of Victor's problem was without a proper diagnosis. It could be his kidneys, bladder, or prostate. I explained to him that urinary tract infections were common in men of his age and burning was a very common symptom. Victor assured me that he did not have any burning sensation, but he agreed to think about having a check-up.

Victor always felt better when I explained things to him and he never doubted me. I had my own medical library and knew my way around *The Merck Manual of Diagnosis and Therapy* – the doctor's bible. I had worked in and managed a drugstore near the corner of Yonge and Bloor streets in Toronto for many years. That was where we met in 1974. I had waved to him as he was walking by the window one day. When I waved a second time he came in and asked me out to dinner.

Victor had a commercial art business not far from where I worked. As it happened, however, his building was closing down and so was the drugstore I worked in. We decided to take advantage of the opportunity this coincidence afforded and agreed to spend the summer at his cottage in Waubeshene, getting to know each other. The rest, as they say, is history. We married, both of us for the second time, and retired to lead a quiet life in the country.

~

After mulling things over for another day, Victor agreed to see a doctor.

I made the appointment for him. "It's settled then!" I said, replacing the receiver. "Dr. Cronk will see you in his office in Belleville on November 12 at 2:00 p.m."

"I can't wait to meet him," Victor said, making a wry face.

After dinner we dressed for our walk down the country road. This was a track, about half a mile long, between two rural roads at the end of our garden. We called it the country road because it didn't have a name. We walked the road, rain or shine, even in blizzards, when cabin fever overcame us and we had to get out for sanity's sake. We would bundle up and brave the elements, returning to the house with leaden legs and frost-tipped eyelashes.

"Come on, Cleo, let's go."

Halfway down the road we stopped at the marsh. Victor called it the swamp but I preferred to call it the marsh. "'Swamp' makes me think of monsters lurking there," I said, my eyes scanning the stagnant water for signs of movement. A few times we had seen beavers. Blue herons made their nests in the tall deadwood.

Beyond the marsh, the woods came to an abrupt end on the edge of a golden cornfield. Every time we went out, we looked past the cornfield to the horizon to see what Mother Nature had painted, and every time it was a different picture. Victor had captured the scene on canvas a few times when the light was just right, painting the purple and bronze hues with deft strokes of his brush and palette knife. Once we saw a young fawn standing in the long corn. It stood so still that it seemed as if it were mesmerized. As we gazed in admiration she suddenly sprang up and with a few graceful leaps was out of sight in seconds.

When we reached the end of the road we turned around and walked down the opposite side so as not to miss anything. Once Victor spotted a weather-monitoring device dangling from a tall tree but it was too high for us to retrieve it. Another time I was startled to find a small alabaster doll's hand reaching out from under a pine tree.

Friends visiting from Toronto would ask us if we were not bored by country life and we would honestly answer no. There was much to do, looking after the property, the lawns and gardens. All needed constant attention. Victor played golf at the local club and there were shopping trips to Peterborough, Belleville, and Toronto, and a yearly motor trip through the New England states. In winter Victor skied at the local resorts and took a bigger ski trip to New York State. One year he went to Aspen with a few of his buddies. There was Victor's painting and my writing to pass the hours when the weather was bad. We both loved to cook and eat and work the effects off by cutting wood for the two fieldstone fireplaces, one at each end of the house. We also did a fair amount of snowshoeing in winter, traversing ground – especially wetlands – that we could not cover in summer.

Victor became a productive oil artist. He turned out at least two paintings a week, which left little time for boredom.

Towards the end of our walks he would often stop in his tracks and look at me with a mischievous grin. "Race you," he would say, and then he was off and over the fence leaving me behind with the two cats. Pierre and Bebe refused to lower their dignity by chasing after Cleo. I would make a feeble attempt to pursue him.

"I hate running," I would say when I did catch up with him. "You know that. I always feel that my liver is bouncing against my lungs when I run."

"Come here, you Glace Bay kid," he would say, teasing me. "I'm going to kiss you all over and make it better." Then he would chase me around the garden. "Oh, you can run when you want to," he would say, laughing, as Cleo and the two cats joined in the fun.

~

The day of the appointment was beautiful, warm and sunny, more like September than November. It was a good forty-minute drive to Belleville. We both felt the strain caused by Victor's apprehension.

"Hey, Vitts, do you remember the duck we rescued from that vicious dog somewhere along this road a few years ago?"

"I remember very well," he replied. "We took her to the vet

in Trenton. You named her Buddy. You were heartbroken when she didn't make it," he said, patting my knee.

"I would have kept her, you know, and we would have found a mate for her," I said. "I wonder how many ducks we would have had by now." I laughed. The duck story reminded me of the time I wanted to keep a baby skunk that took up residence under the canoe, much to the surprise of the two cats, who kept their distance, and Cleo, who barked at it. Finally Victor, dressed in his ski suit, goggles and gloves, and all the protective gear he could put on, shooed the little skunk down the path towards the woods. I faithfully placed food scraps and fruit on the path for the next few weeks until I felt the skunk was grown and out of danger. One day Victor saw the skunk from the window in the studio and told me that the little one had indeed grown up.

Because she continued to stick around for some time we named her Honey. Whenever we asked Cleo, "Where's Honey?" she would woof and look towards the path.

"We've had a lot of wonderful experiences living in the country, haven't we, Vitts?"

"You could write a book, sweetheart," he said, patting my knee as he always did when he was driving and wanted to confirm something or reassure me.

Victor made a right turn off the highway into the parking lot of the Belleville Mall. Before I could say anything he jumped out of the car and opened the passenger-side door for me. "There's no need for you to come, sweetheart," he said. "Why don't you look around and buy something nice for yourself and I'll meet you at the coffee shop in the mall in, say, about an hour?"

He went on to the doctor's office on his own.

"Oh! You're an artist," the receptionist said. "What kind of painting do you do?"

"I'm a landscape artist, but I do some portraits," he replied. He never liked talking about his work but talked readily to others about theirs.

Almost immediately a nurse led him into Dr. Cronk's office.

Victor liked the doctor immediately. A little on the frail side, Dr. Cronk was about his own age, lean and blue-eyed with a warm smile.

Victor noticed photos of the doctor with friends dressed in ski gear.

"Are you a skier, Mr. Newton?" Dr. Cronk asked, following Victor's gaze.

"Yes, I am. I was in Aspen last season. Was this picture taken there?" he asked. "It looks familiar."

"It was indeed," the doctor replied. He looked down at the forms the nurse had placed on his desk. "What can I do for you, Mr. Newton?"

Victor explained that because he would soon be sixty, he thought it would be a good idea to have a check-up. He mentioned that, other than a few extra night-time trips to the bathroom, he was feeling pretty good.

"Any burning or pain when you pass your urine?"

"No, not at all."

"Trouble getting started?"

"Yes, I would say so." Victor changed positions in the chair.

"How many times do you get up at night?"

"Oh, I would say three, sometimes four." Victor was feeling uneasy and he sighed aloud.

"All right, Mr. Newton. Why don't I examine you? You can go into the examining room. My nurse will look after you and I'll be in shortly."

The nurse asked Victor to remove his clothes and put on a paper gown with the opening at the back, then left the room.

The examination was routine but thorough. "Let's see, you weigh 175 pounds and you are five feet and ten and a half inches tall, a good weight and height for your medium frame," the doctor told him. "Your blood pressure is a little low but that's okay. You have exceptional circulation in those legs. All that skiing, eh?" He smiled. "There's a little heart murmur. We can set up a stress test for you at the hospital and an ECG. I don't think it's anything to worry about, but we want to make sure. Now, this is the part you won't like, but it is necessary." He pulled on a latex glove and reached for a lubricating cream. "I want to check your prostate and to do that I have to insert my finger into your rectum. That way I can feel your prostate through the wall of your bowel. Now, I want you to lie on your side and bring your knees up. That's it, Mr. Newton."

He's right, Victor thought, *I don't like it. It's damned uncomfortable and embarrassing, but if it has to be done, let's get it over with.*

Dr. Cronk probed the wall of Victor's bowel and easily found the prostate. What he found next disheartened him: a well-defined nodule about the size of a large pea, hard and foreign. He knew only too well what it meant. "Okay, Mr. Newton, you can get dressed now and I'll see you in my office."

So far, so good, Victor thought as he sat in the black leather chair and waited for Dr. Cronk to look up from the file in front of him.

"Mr. Newton," he said slowly, "you have a nodule, a growth on your prostate, and I'm sorry to say I strongly suspect it to be malignant. Now, these cancers caught early enough are highly treatable," he said, noticing the colour drain from Victor's face. "They're doing marvellous things with radiation these days. A friend of mine and fellow physician is having radiation treatment for prostate cancer and he's doing very well. As a matter of fact, that's him in the photo, the one on the left."

Victor glanced at the three grinning skiers. "Will I still be able to ski?" he asked, feeling a little foolish.

"Certainly," the doctor said with relief. He was never sure how a patient would react when given the news that he had a potentially fatal disease, especially cancer. "I would like you to see a Dr. Hambley in Peterborough. He is a urologist. He'll look after you. My nurse will set up the appointment for you."

They both stood up and shook hands across the desk. Dr. Cronk walked him to the door. "Goodbye, Mr. Newton, and good luck."

Victor got into the car with a blank mind. He sat there for a few minutes as if stunned. He tried to remember all that the doctor had told him. *Damn!* he thought. *Audrey will want to know exactly what the doctor said. Well, it'll come to me.* He started the car and drove to the mall.

"I just don't know how he can say it's a malignancy without a biopsy," I said when I heard the news. My voice was pitched higher than normal.

"He wants me to see a Dr. Hambley in Peterborough who will do the biopsy just to make sure." Victor handed me the appointment card. "But that's not for another two weeks, unless there is a cancellation, in which case they'll call me."

"Are you sure he said radiation, Victor?"

"I'm sure," he replied. "Look, let's not talk about it until we know more. No sense driving ourselves crazy."

That evening we sat at the dining-room table holding hands over the beautiful lace tablecloth his mother had made long years before. The house was deathly silent. Cleo and the two cats were unusually quiet as though they, too, sensed that things were not quite right.

Victor looked at me and narrowed his eyes. "Vood you lak to call up somboody from de spirit vorld?" he asked. We both broke into laughter. He knew when and how to make me laugh, pulling a funny face sometimes after the most heated argument. I always fell for it.

~

We had been living on a modest family inheritance which Victor had invested in the stock market. The market had its ups and downs but nothing to cause him any major concern. But the day after his appointment with Dr. Cronk, Victor received a phone call from his broker.

"My God, what is it?" I asked when he put down the phone. "You're as white as a sheet!"

"The market has crashed. We've lost half our money. Frank said things are crazy at the market and they might get worse."

"Victor dear, take the rest of it out, now, before we lose it all."

"I can't do that," he said, pacing back and forth. "What if the market recovers?"

"What if it doesn't?" I countered.

"I'll call Frank before the market closes and see how things are before I make any hard decisions."

By late afternoon the market was still falling and with it went most of what we had left. Sleep did not come easily to either of us that night as we tossed and turned and Victor made the usual half-dozen trips to the bathroom.

We finally fell asleep only to be jarred awake by the ringing of the telephone. It was Frank. Things had worsened.

"Do you want me to pull out now, Vic?"

"Not yet," Victor replied. "I think I'll come over to the office now." He drove to the brokerage house in Peterborough alone. He didn't want me with him. He was upset and having trouble thinking clearly.

I, too, was sick with worry. I walked back and forth along the country road so many times that even Cleo refused to accompany me. I hopped over the fence and ran through the garden when I saw the car pull into the driveway. I knew when I saw him, standing beside the car, his arms hanging heavy at his sides, that it was all over. There would be no more checking the business section of *The Globe and Mail* for the latest stock market results.

"I wasn't the only one to lose everything. Frank said there was a suicide. A lot of people were completely wiped out."

"How awful. Don't worry, sweetheart, we'll get it all straightened out," I said soothingly.

"Don't you understand?" he said, taking me by the shoulders.

"We're broke and I have cancer. How are we going to straighten that out?"

I was about to cry but swallowed hard instead. "I'm a survivor," I said. "We'll get through this and we'll be all right. I promise you."

"Come here, you Glace Bay kid," he said. He held me close. "Thank God I've got you. That's all that really matters to me."

Later, when we were able to put things into perspective, Victor called the bank manager in Campbellford and asked him if he would carry us until we sold the house. Next he called his brother Tom.

Tom, five years his senior, had an accounting firm in Kingston. When tax time rolled around Victor would gather up his receipts and any suspicious-looking papers, place them in a large envelope, and mail them to Tom. He always sighed with relief when a neat brown envelope came back with a copy of his tax return and a modest bill. "Done for another year," Victor would announce with a grin. Now he told his brother the whole unfortunate story.

Tom agreed to sign a bank loan and the bank agreed to extend the loan if necessary until the house was sold. The real estate market was at a standstill. We would have to be patient, but at least we were secure for a while. In the meantime, Victor had to see Dr. Hambley in Peterborough.

Treatment

The Most Common Diagnostic Tests for Prostate Cancer

Digital Rectal Examination (DRE)

Most men dread this examination, but it's simple and quick, and should be a part of the regular medical check-up of any man over forty years of age. The doctor places a gloved finger, to which he has applied a lubricating cream, into the rectum and feels the prostate through the wall of the bowel. He checks for a nodule, a lump, or anything unusual. If the doctor finds something abnormal he will order further tests.

Prostate-Specific Antigen (PSA)

A positive result from this simple blood test may point towards the possibility of a prostate gland disorder. Prostate-specific antigen is a protein produced only by the prostate gland. A high level of this protein can indicate a number of disorders of the prostate gland, including prostate cancer and benign prostatic hyperplasia (or BPH – an enlarged prostate). This test has largely replaced the acid phosphatese test which was used to diagnose prostate problems when Victor was first examined for prostate cancer. Some doctors feel that the PSA test is the best early indicator of the presence of cancer in the prostate gland. It is not, however, infallible.

Transrectal Ultrasound (TRUS)

The principle of ultrasound is that sound waves are directed at a specific part of the body. Because different tissues and organs are more or less dense, the waves either bounce or go through, and the readings picked up by the ultrasound scanner reflect these variations in density.

When ultrasound is used for the diagnosis of prostate conditions, a probe is inserted into the rectum, aimed at the prostate, and an ultrasound picture is recorded. The resulting ultrasound image may indicate the presence of a tumour, its size, and the extent to which it has spread. Ultrasound cannot, however, distinguish between a malignant and a benign tumour.

In addition to its usefulness in detecting a tumour, the transrectal ultrasound may also be used by the doctor to guide the needle into the prostate while he performs a biopsy.

The first two tests (DRE and PSA) may be conducted or ordered more or less routinely by a family doctor. If both are positive, the doctor is likely to refer the patient to a urologist, a specialist in the treatment of urinary disorders, including disorders of the prostate. The urologist may repeat both tests and order, in addition, the transrectal ultrasound. If all of these tests are positive, that is, the patient has a suspicious lump, an elevated PSA, and an abnormal transrectal ultrasound, the doctor will almost certainly schedule a biopsy. However, in most cases a highly elevated PSA alone may be enough to go to biopsy. Although PSA is by far the best marker for detecting prostate cancer it is not perfect. It sometimes produces false positive and false negative results. These drawbacks are currently being investigated.

Biopsy

A biopsy is the surgical removal of a piece of tissue so that it can be viewed under a microscope. This procedure is done to either confirm or exclude the presence of a malignancy. The biopsy may be either transrectal (through the rectum) or transperineal (through the perineum). In the transrectal biopsy procedure (which is performed without using a local anaesthetic) a needle is placed directly into the prostate gland through the rectum. In the transperineal biopsy (which usually requires an anaesthetic), the doctor pushes a very fine needle through the perineum, which is the space between the scrotum and the anus. Some doctors prefer the perineal approach because it is thought to be the less painful of the two, but because the transperineal biopsy yields only a small quantity of prostatic tissue, the procedure may have to be repeated, while the transrectal approach usually produces an adequate sample. The transrectal biopsy is more commonly used. In either case, the cells taken from the prostate are examined by another medical specialist, a pathologist, who reports on the presence or absence of disease in the sample.

The biopsy is normally performed in hospital on an out-patient basis.

Prostate Cancer

The biopsy is usually considered to be conclusive. That is, the result of the biopsy will be a definite diagnosis. In the event that the diagnosis is cancer, further tests will be called for to determine how widespread the cancer is. These additional tests may include a bone scan. In this test a low-dosage radioactive substance is injected into a vein in the arm. The substance then collects in the bones where a scanner pinpoints areas of abnormal bone activity and an X-ray image is produced. The test is painless and is usually done to determine if cancer has spread to the pelvic bone and the spine. Another test may involve magnetic resonance imaging (MRI), which is the latest thing in medical diagnostic X-ray scanners that can be directed at specific areas of concern. The kinds of tests that are employed vary according to what the doctor requires and the stage of cancer.

The Stages of Prostate Cancer

There are two well-known staging systems for prostate cancer. They are the International Union Against Cancer (UICC) system and the American Urologic System. The American Urologic System is less precise than the other system but is easier to understand and is probably adequate for present purposes. According to this system, there are four distinct stages of prostate cancer: A, B, C, and D. The tests ordered by the urologist are intended to determine how far the cancer has spread, which then indicates the stage of the disease.

Stage A

There are usually no symptoms at this stage. Cancer at this stage is usually found by chance, perhaps during surgery for another problem.

Stage B

The cancer is still confined to the prostate gland and has not invaded any surrounding tissue or lymph nodes. At this stage, a tumour or nodule may be felt by the urologist when he conducts a digital rectal examination. Further tests – PSA, ultrasound, and a biopsy – may then be ordered. The results of these tests will confirm a positive or negative diagnosis.

Stage C

The malignant tumour has now spread beyond the confines of the prostate gland. At this stage the growth may be putting pressure on the urethra, causing problems with passing urine. These symptoms, which have been listed in the section "Symptoms and Diagnosis" – getting up at night, trouble getting started, a stream that stops and starts or dribbles – are likely to alert the individual to the problem. At this stage there may also be pain in the area of the prostate gland.

Stage D

The tumour has now spread, or metastasized, to the surrounding lymph nodes. Over time, other parts of the body may become involved. Common sites are the bones, especially in the spine, and organs such as the lungs and the liver. Stage D is subdivided into stages D1 and D2 according to how far the cancer has spread.

When Victor was diagnosed in 1981, his cancer was discovered to be a Stage D1 tumour: the cancer had invaded the surrounding lymph nodes. He was not in any pain or distress, however, except for the pressure on his urethra, which was alleviated with treatment.

Treatment

Each stage of prostate cancer is treated according to the extent of the disease. The urologist will talk with each patient individually about the treatment suitable for his case. Each case is, of course, different. The range of treatments for prostate cancer include surgery, radiation, and hormone drug therapy. Chemotherapy is now an effective and relatively non-toxic therapy. It is useful for palliative care only.

Possible Treatment at Stages A and B

Radical prostatectomy, the complete surgical removal of the prostate gland, is the usual choice of treatment for early stage cancers in which the tumour is confined to the prostate and there is no evidence of spread to the surrounding lymph nodes and tissue. Some urologists may recommend radiation therapy instead of surgery depending on the patient's age and state of health. However, for older men with good prognostic factors, "watch and wait" is becoming an accepted practice. PSA testing allows for close monitoring with intervention if necessary. A patient who is in his mid-seventies or eighties may have another serious health problem, such as heart disease, in which case a "watch and wait" approach may be recommended as a way of dealing with his prostate cancer. Because it is usually such a slow-growing disease, he is more likely to die with it rather than of it. If there is any doubt about the right treatment in a particular case and the patient is unsure, he can always get another opinion. It is always better to be satisfied that the most appropriate course of action is being pursued before any action is taken.

Possible Treatment at Stage C
When the cancer is in Stage C the malignant tumour is both inside and outside the prostate gland and has invaded the surrounding tissue. Treatment is designed to control the spread. Radiation therapy and/or hormonal drug therapy is the usual choice of treatment. Hormonal therapy in Stage C may include an orchiectomy, which is the complete surgical removal of the testicles – castration. Orchiectomy is advised in some cases because the testicles produce the male hormone testosterone and it has been found that the presence of testosterone causes prostate cancer to grow and spread more rapidly than it would otherwise. There are also effective non-surgical alternatives to orchiectomy. Depending on how far the cancer has advanced and the individual needs of the patient, the choice of surgical or non-surgical treatment may be left up to him. Again, there are no hard and fast rules.

Possible Treatment at Stage D
In Stage D cancer of the prostate, orchiectomy is strongly recommended. Victor's case was, in this respect, an exception: because radiation therapy was so successful, an orchiectomy was neither performed nor advised. Most men cringe at the mere mention of this procedure, and not without reason: it inevitably means the loss of sexual function. There are a number of myths

about the procedure. Some men believe, for example, that castration is the complete surgical removal of the scrotum (the sac that contains the testicles); this is not so. The surgeon makes a small incision in the scrotum, and removes the two small glands, the testicles, and then stitches the opening together again. The scrotum remains. The procedure is a simple one involving a stay in hospital of about a day, two at most.

Orchiectomy is more likely to be performed on an older than a younger man. Hormone therapy, using drugs, is a kind of medical castration. In other words, the production of testosterone is suppressed using drugs instead of surgery. Both medical castration, by hormone therapy, and surgical castration inevitably result in impotence and the loss of libido – the sexual urge. Orchiectomy produces hot flashes, which diminish in time. The procedure is undoubtedly a drastic one, but the alternative is more drastic still: thousands of men are living longer lives thanks to this surgery.

A Reminder

As indicated in the disclaimer at the front of this book, the information given here is general and, to a degree, simplified. Armed with this information, the reader should be better equipped to understand what his doctor tells him about his particular case and to ask questions about it. This information is not a substitute for the advice of a doctor who is familiar with a patient's medical history and who has full knowledge of the range of options appropriate to his case.

Possible Side Effects of Cancer Treatments

Every treatment for prostate cancer has some side effects. For the most part they diminish as the patient's body adjusts to the treatment and heals.

Side Effects of Surgery

Side effects of surgery may be mild or severe. Some of the most common side effects experienced by patients following radical prostatectomy are impotence, incontinence, fatigue, and, in some cases, bloating of the abdomen due to fluid retention. Prostate cancer that has metastasized is very rarely treated with surgery. The cancer almost always goes to the bone and is usually treated with radiation therapy to reduce the pain.

Fatigue is another common side effect of prostate – or any – surgery and it may be several months before the patient regains his strength and feels his old self again.

Side Effects of Radiation Therapy

Most men go through radiation therapy with few troublesome side effects. Others suffer from one or more debilitating side effects, such as rectal irritation, diarrhoea, and a sensitive urinary tract. In some cases radiation to the prostate can cause painless bleeding to the lower bowel. This is almost always harmless but can be quite frightening at first. In any case, you should report any bleeding or other unusual side effects to your doctor and radiation technician.

For those who find the treatment hard to take, there are ways to relieve some of the discomfort. The patient's doctor and radiation technician may provide information or pamphlets about a particular treatment. The patient should never worry in silence. Doctors will explain everything, but sometimes they have to be asked.

Most side effects disappear after a few weeks. About half of men treated lose sexual function at least temporarily.

Side Effects of Hormone Drug Therapy

When Victor was treated with hormone drug therapy he suffered unpleasant side effects. He developed painful swelling of his breasts. He also suffered from hot flashes similar to those women sometimes experience in menopause. Some men become very emotional and cry easily, for example, until they adjust to the hormones. These side effects are caused by the female hormones, including estrogen, in the hormone drug therapy. Now, ten years later, there are newer drugs with fewer side effects. Nevertheless, fatigue continues to be a common side effect of this treatment.

Sexual Dysfunction

Impotence (the inability to get an erection) and loss of libido (lack of sexual desire) are major concerns for the prostate cancer sufferer. Surgery for both benign and malignant prostate cancer can significantly affect sexual functioning. Orchiectomy, hormone therapy, and radiation therapy may have similar results. In many other cases, however, where the treatment is less drastic, impotence may be a temporary condition caused by the overwhelming emotional impact of the disease. The disruption of everyday life can be a strong influence on a man's ability to perform sexually and the cancer sufferer's life is invariably disrupted. A man who has to deal with anxiety, depression, and fear needs time to recover and relax.

When Victor became impotent while on hormone therapy in 1982, he was very angry. He muttered about it under his breath and even cursed the doctors. Then he did something I never dreamed he would do – he shut me out. He moved to the far side of the bed and refused to talk about his concerns. It was some time before we were able to communicate again. He told me then that he had been afraid I would not love him any more. After I reassured him of my love, he welcomed me back into his arms where I belonged. From that time on I encouraged Victor to talk about his feelings.

If you are experiencing problems with impotence, don't withdraw into yourself, and don't worry in silence. Talk to your partner. And ask your doctor – he or she understands and will answer all your questions. Remember, your urologist has studied this disease and he deals with men in your situation every day. It's always a good idea, incidentally, to make a list of the more important questions you want to ask before you go into the doctor's office.

If you would like to investigate the newer techniques to restore sexual functioning, such as penile implants and mechanical devices such as pumps and vacuum constrictors, discuss the subject with your urologist. He will have the latest information and will suggest the best choice in your case.

Incontinence

Although surgical techniques and treatment for prostate cancer continue to improve, incontinence (loss of voluntary bladder control) can still be a problem. The discomfort, inconvenience, and fear of losing urine in a public place can cause an otherwise extroverted individual to become introverted very quickly. That, of course, need not be the case. More than ten million men and women in the United States and Canada suffer from some degree of incontinence. It is a common problem and there is a lot of help available. Your doctor will discuss various ways to deal with it. Absorbent pads, which are easy to use and readily found in all drugstores, are a common choice. Don't be afraid to talk with your urologist about this. He understands that you may be embarrassed and can advise you on the best approach to managing your own particular degree of incontinence. He will also inform you of some exercises that you may be able to do to strengthen the muscles around your bladder.

The biopsy was to be performed at the Peterborough Civic Hospital. I didn't meet the doctor at the hospital. I sat in the waiting room and turned pages of outdated magazines while I tried to imagine what Victor was going through.

An elderly lady with blue-grey hair slapped a magazine down on the glass-topped table, making everyone jump. "I wouldn't read that trash," she announced in a huff.

"Mrs. Newton! Mrs. Victor Newton!"

"Yes, I'm here." I reached for my coat and followed the nurse.

"You can take your husband home now," she said. "Dr. Hambley will see him in his office at the medical centre next Friday, and by the way, Mr. Newton has had a light anaesthetic. He is awake; however, we do not want him to drive."

Before I could reply, I saw Victor walking towards me looking a little dazed and pale. I led him out of the hospital to the parking lot. It had been snowing.

"Look, Vitts, the first snowfall. Take a deep breath, sweetheart." I opened the door on the passenger's side for him.

"What are you doing?" he asked, a little surprised.

"I'm driving us home. Don't worry, I'll be careful," I said. I took a deep breath myself. I did not usually drive. I had been a nervous driver and never really liked it.

At home, I helped him out of his clothes and saw the blood on his boxer shorts right away. I got a warm wash cloth and wiped the blood away. I brought him a cup of hot soup and kissed his cool forehead. "It's only 1:00 p.m., we didn't do too badly, Vitts. Now I want you to get some rest."

He slept soundly for a few hours and was surprisingly alert when he joined me in the family room. I had a good blaze going in the fireplace and spaghetti sauce simmering on the stove in the kitchen. Pierre and Bebe were curled up together on the sofa while snow continued to fall softly outside. It fluttered down through the birch and maple trees on the other side of the big picture window. Victor opened the door and let Cleo in for her afternoon visit. After much woofing and tail-wagging she settled down with her head between her paws, raising and lowering her huge brown eyes each time we spoke and sighing loudly with contentment.

"Can you remember what the doctor did?" I asked, sensing that he was ready to talk about it.

"It hurt like a son-of-a-bitch, even with the anaesthetic. He put something up through my penis and had a look at my bladder. I think he took a piece of my prostate. Worst bloody thing I ever had to endure," he said with a shudder.

"Oh, you poor angel." I held him close. "Does it hurt now?"

"It stung when I went to the bathroom a few minutes ago.

33

Look, I don't want you getting upset. I'm fine now. Let's have dinner, it smells good." He was hungry. *That's always a good sign,* I thought, piling our plates with spaghetti.

One week later we were in Dr. Hambley's office in Peterborough.

"Mr. Newton, good to see you. How are you feeling today?" Dr. Hambley shook Victor's hand. "I see you are an artist. What kind of painting do you do?"

"Landscapes and some portraits," Victor replied.

"I had an aunt who was a pretty good artist." The doctor held his pen at both ends between his fingertips.

Victor listened politely. Almost everybody, like the doctor, knew someone who painted a little.

Small talk over, Victor turned the conversation to the real reason he was sitting in the doctor's office instead of at home in Warkworth painting snowy landscapes. "Would you mind if I ask my wife to come in, Doctor?" he asked. "She likes to know everything and I won't remember."

"By all means," the doctor replied. "I was going to suggest it myself."

"Dr. Hambley, my wife, Audrey."

We smiled at each other, shook hands, then Victor and I settled into the big comfortable chairs and waited for the doctor to speak.

"You have cancer, Mr. Newton, cancer of the prostate." Silence filled the room like a darkening fog. I thought of Dr. Cronk. *He really knows his business. He was right.* Victor and I stared at the doctor waiting for his next words, waiting for a lifeline.

"We can't be sure to what extent the cancer has spread, or if it has." The doctor looked at Victor and then at me. "I want you to see another urologist, Dr. Farrow, at the Toronto General Hospital. We didn't get a good biopsy; however, there is a strong possibility that the cancer is contained to the prostate. If that is the case, Dr. Farrow will want to operate and remove the entire prostate gland. If the cancer has spread he will not remove it. Once the cancer is in the lymphatic system there is no use in removing the prostate gland. In which case, Dr. Farrow will probably want to treat you with hormones to control the spread."

"Since you didn't get a good biopsy, isn't it possible that it isn't cancer?" I asked, my tone pleading.

"I doubt it, Mrs. Newton. You see, we did a blood test called the acid phosphatase test. This test measures an enzyme secreted by the prostate gland. When the level of this enzyme is elevated, coupled with the positive findings of the digital rectal exam, we can be pretty sure of an existing cancer. Dr. Farrow will do a complete series of tests and another biopsy before he decides on what course he will take.

"Now I want you to give me a urine sample, Mr. Newton." The doctor gestured towards the bathroom.

Getting up from the chair Victor took the container from the doctor and met my eyes for a moment. The corners of his mouth turned up in a weak smile. I sensed he wanted to take me in his arms and say, "I'm sorry for bursting our wonderful bubble."

~

A week before Christmas we heard from Dr. Farrow's office. An appointment was made for January 2, Victor's sixtieth birthday. We were relieved that it was after Christmas. We didn't want to spoil anyone's holiday spirit with talk of cancer. We had put off telling any of the family, except Tom, about our misfortunes.

It was hard to feel Christmassy so we didn't try. Although money was tight, we managed to buy a few gifts for Victor's daughters, Sandy and Laurie. The girls were spending Christmas with their mother, and my son, Rob, had made no bones about his plans for the holidays. He informed me he would be spending them with his friends in Toronto.

Christmas Day was not entirely uneventful. We were awakened by Cleo's anguished bark early in the morning.

"Oh no," I moaned, burying myself deeper in the warm duvet.

"She just wants her Christmas presents," Victor said. Wrapping his old terrycloth robe around himself, he let the big dog into the house. "Good grief! Audrey, come and see Cleo."

Cleo sheepishly hung her head as we scolded her. "Where have you been? What have you done? You bad dog."

The big Newfie was stuck like a pincushion with more than two dozen porcupine quills. Victor got the pliers and I soothed and comforted the trembling dog who yelped with each pull of the hooked, needlelike quills. When we thought we had got them all we discovered another one way down the back of her throat.

"Looks like she tried to swallow the whole creature," I said, rubbing an antibiotic ointment onto the dog's tender nose. We continued to scold her. Cleo covered her eyes with her big paws and sighed loudly before she mercifully fell asleep.

Around noon the girls called to wish us Merry Christmas. Although we tried to sound cheerful, the atmosphere hung heavy and sad. Sensing a little activity was called for, I suggested a brisk walk down the country road and a frolic in the deep snow followed by hot chocolate and a big bowl of buttery popcorn. Our spirits seemed to lift as the day wore on.

A few days later, Victor's sister Anne called with an invitation to join her and her daughter Molly for lunch at her apartment in Toronto. I welcomed a change of scene and accepted.

"The weather was fine and the drive to Toronto was pleasant. Not too much traffic," Victor told Anne as she kissed us both and took our coats. It was the first time I had seen him relating to other people since his diagnosis.

It seemed odd that everything was so normal. *This is my husband,* I thought, *this handsome, healthy-looking man with the grey hair, green eyes, and pink complexion. This man with the wonderful quick laugh, this distinguished gentleman in his navy-blue suit, white shirt, and paisley tie. This is my husband and he has cancer.*

Suddenly I was hearing the dreaded word. Molly was talking about a friend who had fought the brave fight with cancer, lost her breast and her hair and died courageously with her family at her side.

"Don't you think Victor looks wonderful?" I blurted out, rising to my feet. "We really must be going. We don't want to get caught in heavy traffic."

Anne looked surprised. As we were leaving we heard Molly say, "What the hell was that all about?"

"I'm sorry, Victor, but when Molly was talking about her

friend, I thought I would break apart. I just had to get out of there."

"It's all right, sweetheart. They'll know soon enough and they'll understand." He patted my knee and turned onto the highway towards home.

~

A week later Victor and I were in Dr. Farrow's waiting room, which he shared with two other prominent urologists at the Toronto General Hospital. I recognized another tall, blue-eyed, blond doctor who had been on television several times talking about kidney transplants. The room was full. The majority of patients were men.

After the routine filling out of forms, we were ushered into the doctor's office. Dr. Farrow introduced himself and waved Victor into the examining room.

"I'm going to examine your prostate, Mr. Newton. No need to take everything off, just your pants and underwear will do. Now if you will get up on the table and lie on your side, that's it." Victor felt the doctor's finger, probing inside his rectum.

God almighty, I hate this, he said to himself, feeling a rage welling up.

"Okay, Mr. Newton, you can get dressed now." The doctor removed his latex gloves and left him alone. Victor returned to the outer office where I was waiting. I noticed the strain on his face. The digital exam always upset him. His rectum would be irritated for the rest of the day.

Dr. Farrow returned to the office. I was reminded of the Great Gatsby when I looked at him. Like Gatsby, he was a handsome man with fine features and straight hair combed back. I guessed that he was probably in his early fifties. The doctor with his hands, thumbs out, in the pockets of his white surgical coat looked at both of us for a long moment. He sat down and looked over the papers on his desk.

"I see Dr. Hambley did not get a good biopsy. However, your acid phosphatase blood test was quite high. I would like to admit you to the hospital here and do another biopsy. After that we will operate with the intention of removing the entire prostate gland. Before we do, we will check the lymph nodes and if any cancer cells are found, we will not remove the gland; instead, we will treat the cancer with hormone therapy."

"What kind of hormones?" I asked, wide-eyed.

"Diethylstilbestrol. This drug slows the production of testosterone, the male hormone produced by the testicles. Testosterone causes the cancer to grow more rapidly."

"What about the operation?" Victor interjected. "Dr. Hambley said it may be rough."

"Well, I don't know of any operation that is pleasant," Dr. Farrow replied. "No doubt it is a rough operation; however, it is a cure. Consider the alternative. What would you choose? There are side effects," he continued. "You will be impotent and possibly lose bladder control. There are exercises you can do after surgery to strengthen the bladder with good results, but that's a long way down the road."

"Are there any side effects with the hormone treatment?" I asked, shifting in my chair.

"Yes, you will still be impotent, Mr. Newton. The diethylstilbestrol stops the production of the male hormone testosterone. Testosterone is responsible for the sex drive. Do you understand?" He was sitting on the edge of his desk with his arms crossed.

"What are my chances?" Victor asked, looking strained and pale.

The doctor was on his feet now, leaning over his desk, drawing on a sheet of paper. "This is the prostate gland wrapped around the urethra. As you can see, it is about the size of a walnut," he said. "If we remove the gland it will be because the cancer is contained, and you will be cured. You can expect to live a full life span, barring any fatal diseases or accidents. If the cancer has spread beyond the prostate, you are looking at from two to five years."

"When will you do the biopsy?" I asked, reaching for the illustrated piece of paper.

"As soon as we can get your husband admitted and book the surgery," Dr. Farrow replied.

He looked at his watch. "My secretary will be in touch with you," he said, shaking Victor's hand. "The surgery should be soon, within a few weeks," he added. He walked us to the door, glanced at his watch again and at the crowded waiting room.

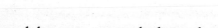

A week later we received a letter from Dr. Farrow's office with a set of admission and X-ray acquisition forms. The surgery was scheduled for January 18, 1982, at the Toronto General Hospital.

I had not said or done anything to mark Victor's birthday. Somehow it seemed insensitive to wish him a happy birthday in our present situation, and yet it was a milestone.

"You know, Vitts, now that you are the big six-o, I love you more than ever," I said. "You'll make it to the over-seventy, ski free club, I promise." I put my arms around him and held him tight.

"You sweetheart," he said. "You always make me feel better. You really think I'll make it to seventy?"

"I absolutely believe it, Vitts," I replied seriously. "You must believe it, too. You must!"

"You know," he said, "this is the first year I haven't skied since I was fourteen years old."

The snow fell beyond the picture window. It was falling steadily on the Northumberland hills, the Warkworth pond, and the little graveyard on the edge of town. Victor thought of the people he had come to know in the village who were now resting in the graveyard. Jim, the happy-go-lucky clerk who had worked in the liquor store, suffered a massive heart attack. Jackie, a sunny sixteen-year-old, had been tragically killed in a car accident on her prom night. Old Percy, the man we bought our house from. They had all been full of life and laughter. Now they were asleep in death, and the snow fell quietly on their graves.

The days passed quickly. There was much to do and little time to reflect on the magnitude of what lay ahead of us. It was time to call the family and inform them of Victor's cancer. He asked me to call. He could not bring himself to speak the words.

I called the girls first. When I did not get an answer, I called his former wife, Barb.

Upon hearing the news Barb offered to tell the girls herself. Her own husband, a heavy smoker, had died of lung cancer two years after they were married.

"You know, that's exactly what happened here," she said, referring to her late husband's cancer, without actually saying the dreaded word.

"Not exactly," I said, "Victor is not in a late stage of cancer and we expect a full recovery after surgery."

"Well, don't expect too much, it might be quick," she added. Her own husband had died within weeks of his diagnosis.

Next, I called Victor's brother Chuck and his sisters, Marg and Anne. They were older than Victor and were quite alarmed by the news. I told them that we had talked to Tom, and asked them to inform the rest of the family, and soon the telephone was ringing.

Ronnie, Victor's nephew, a gregarious fellow, asked, "What the hell is this about, Uncle Vic?"

When the calls were finished, I felt incredibly tired. We both fell asleep, quickly and gratefully.

~

"This is your locker, you can put your things in here, Mr. Newton." The nurse sat in a chair beside the bed with her pen and forms ready. "We have to fill these out," she said. "Dr. Shum will be in later to see you. He's Dr. Farrow's assistant."

When she had gone, I checked out the locker and bathroom, while Victor emptied the contents of his bag onto the bed.

"I knew bloody well I'd forget something," he said irritably. "My nail scissors."

"I'll buy new ones," I said. "There's a gift shop downstairs, I'm sure they'll have them."

I sat on the edge of the bed. "I wonder who your roommate is, Vitts." There was another bed next to his, presently unoccupied. Then I said, "They'll be coming soon to take a blood sample. Don't you think you should change into your pyjamas?"

He didn't want to. "What the hell, I guess I have no choice," he said, grumbling.

We were both downhearted and tired. We worried about leaving the animals boarding at the vet's in Trenton. We had never before left them for more than a week; now it would be at least two. The cats would be okay, but Cleo was a big dog, accustomed to being outdoors all day. We also worried about leaving the house in the middle of winter.

"What if the pipes freeze, and what if the real estate people try to get us?" Victor said.

"I've taken care of that, Vitts, I gave them Rob's number. They'll call if they have an interested buyer. Rob will let me know and the pipes should be okay with the heat on low."

A plump, cheery nurse rustled into the room. "I've come to take your blood, Mr. Newton," she said as she tied a rubber tourniquet around his upper arm.

Minutes later another nurse placed a thermometer in his mouth and proceeded to take his blood pressure.

I walked to the other side of the room to the window next to the empty bed, noticing the books and flowers.

Just then a stocky man in his mid-sixties came into the room wearing a ruby-red velvet robe over grey silk pyjamas. His hands were thrust deep into the pockets. He offered his hand to Victor. "How do you do? My name is Vince Gabriele."

"Vic Newton. This is my wife, Audrey."

Vince shuffled to his side of the room and began an exchange of "getting to know you" small talk. Victor was a people person and he liked Vince right away. The conversation soon became animated and punctuated with laughter.

Victor was the first to ask the inevitable question. "So, what brings you here, Vince?" He tried to sound nonchalant.

"Oh, nothing serious," Vince replied, straightening the sheets on his bed. "I'm having my prostate operated on in the morning. They say it's enlarged. I should be out of here in a few days. I'd better be out in a few days," he added emphatically. "I've got contracts to make good on. You know how it is when the boss is away, nothing gets done. What about you?"

"They're doing a biopsy on my prostate in the morning," Victor furrowed his brow. "I'll know more after that." He didn't tell Vince that he was already slated for major surgery a day after the biopsy. One way or the other he would be opened, his belly slit like a fish, so the surgeon could search for the deadly enemy. Victor had had enough. He didn't want to talk about surgery any more.

Both men felt a sense of relief after clearing the air about their respective medical problems and switched easily to a variety of other subjects. I became restless and suggested a walk around the floor, leaving Vince to his chocolate-box-sized TV.

I didn't expect to see women patients. I knew it was the urology floor and had always associated those kinds of problems with men. Now I was learning.

We passed a girl about twenty years old, who was sitting in a wheelchair. Her skin was greenish grey and she looked very ill and frightened. Her dark eyes met ours, and Victor nodded to her.

Along the way we met a half-dozen older men, all pushing IV poles with catheter bags attached, some half filled with bloody urine, which dripped down tubes that had been inserted through their penises into their bladders.

These men were recovering from surgery. They had undergone a procedure called a transurethral resection of the prostate, otherwise known as a TURP, or as Vince called it, a "ream out." In a few days, most would be at home again, little the worse for wear.

~

"How do you do, Mr. Newton? My name is Dr. Shum. I'm Dr. Farrow's assistant. Have you been drinking lots of fluids?"

"Yes, I have. I was expecting dinner, but not in a glass," Victor said, and laughed lightly.

"Yes. Well, we don't want you eating before surgery. Dr. Farrow will be doing the biopsy about 8:00 in the morning. Now Mr. Newton, I want to explain a few things to you and your wife about the operation. You will have the same procedure here for the biopsy as you did in Peterborough. This will be done to confirm the results of the earlier biopsy. You will then be prepared for major surgery the following day."

Victor and I hung onto every word.

"What is the procedure for the removal of the prostate?" Victor asked.

"Dr. Farrow will open you from the navel to the pubic line.

First he will check the lymph nodes for any spread of the cancer. If cancer cells are found he will abandon the original plan to remove the prostate and close you up again," Dr. Shum replied.

"Why?" I asked.

"Because there is no point in removing the prostate gland if the cancer has spread to the surrounding lymph nodes. Your survival time would not be increased at any rate; however, we would treat the cancer with hormone therapy to check the spread."

Victor and I quietly absorbed this information.

"Look, let's not jump the gun," the doctor said, rising to his feet. "There is a good chance your cancer has not spread, in which case the most you will go through is an operation."

Victor let out a deep sigh and met my anxious stare.

"We have a patient who had this surgery a week ago. You might want to talk to him. His name is Doug Campbell. He's in a private room on the other side of the corridor. He may be able to put your mind at ease. I'll see you tomorrow, Mr. Newton. Good night, Mrs. Newton." Dr. Shum nodded graciously and left the room.

"Okay, sweetheart, I'm on my way," I said, reaching for my coat.

"You be careful," Victor said, adding a new worry to his collection, thinking about me making my way across the city to the apartment where I would be staying with my son, Rob, and his girlfriend, Beth. "Be sure to call the minute you get there," he said, holding my hand as he walked me to the elevator.

"I will and I'll be here first thing in the morning."

Victor kissed me, not wanting to let go. He ran back to the window where he caught sight of me as I made my way through the swirling snow and watched until I turned the corner and disappeared from sight. I did not hear him tapping on the window.

≈

When I saw Rob I sensed right away that something was wrong. I thought he must have been worrying about me until I entered the apartment.

I looked around, astonished. Except for a chair and a mattress, the apartment was empty.

"Beth and I split," Rob said with downcast eyes. "She came with her father while I was at work and cleaned the place out. She took everything." Rob glanced up quickly and waited for me to say something. I sat on the chair and held my head in my hands.

"I can't go into this now, Rob, I just can't."

"I know, Mom. Look, it'll be okay; I'll go out and get some things tomorrow, some necessities. You take the mattress and I'll sleep on the floor tonight."

I lay awake. Rob was fast asleep. His breathing seemed to bounce off the walls and echo in the bare rooms. I thought about Beth. I had liked her very much and after a three-year relationship I had expected Rob and she would marry.

I felt a heavy weariness come over me but suppressed the sobs that strained at my throat. *I have to stay strong and in control for Victor*, I thought, as I felt the room shudder above the rumbling subway below. Freezing rain pelted the window with a vengeance.

Rob took the following day off and was out and back before I finished in the bathroom. He had bought pillows, blankets, cutlery and dishes.

"Here, this is for you." He handed me a mug with little red hearts on it and "MOM" in big letters. I was touched.

"That's sweet, Rob, I'll have my tea in it now." I sipped the hot tea and listened as Rob told me how he had come home early one day to find Beth with another guy. That was a month ago, Rob said, and they had been fighting ever since.

"She told me it was just the one time and asked me to forgive her. I couldn't. I still love her and yet I know it's over. I could never trust her again."

Rob stared down at the floor. I felt his pain but could say nothing. Victor and I never interfered in our children's lives. We gave advice, help, and most of all love, but we did not make judgements.

Finally I spoke. "Well, Rob, if you can't forgive her you'll have to learn how to start over, slowly, one day at a time and it will take time. Separating from someone you love is a kind of death. You'll need to grieve and heal." I kissed him on the forehead. "I have to go. I don't want to worry Victor."

"Say hello for me," Rob said. "I know he doesn't want anyone coming to the hospital for a few days, but I'll be there when he is ready."

Rob walked me to the subway. "See you later, Mom." He turned and walked back towards the apartment. I noticed a slump in his shoulders and my heart ached for him.

~

"Well, look at you, you look fine," I said, as I fell into Victor's waiting arms.

"I am fine, sweetheart, but you look tired. You shouldn't worry so much."

"Well, tell me, how did the biopsy go?" I took a piece of toast from his late breakfast tray.

"Pretty much the same as it did the last time. I saw Dr. Farrow for a few minutes before they put me out. He said that he would see me later today with the results and to explain a few things about the surgery. That's all I know. I'm a little sore. It stings when I pee," he whispered.

"I'm surprised they gave you breakfast when you are scheduled for major surgery tomorrow morning."

"Nothing after 12:00 noon. That's when they start cleaning me out again." Victor rolled his eyes. "Eat the rest of the toast. I saved it for you. I want you to go down to the cafeteria at lunch time and eat a good meal. I don't want my angel getting sick." He seemed to be taking everything in his stride.

I said nothing about Rob and Beth. I absolutely did not want him to suffer any more stress. He had enough to deal with. I looked around the room.

"Vince hasn't come back from the operating room," he said, following my gaze.

"Good! Now I have you all to myself," I said, playfully kissing his mouth and eyelids.

"I love you so much," he said, holding me close. I nestled against his broad chest where I had always felt safe.

"Oh God, now what?" Victor groaned. An orderly carrying a stainless steel tray came towards the bed.

"Hi, Mr. Newton. My name is Jerry and I'm going to prep you for tomorrow's surgery."

I moved quickly out of the way, winking at Victor. "I'll be right here, Vitts." I picked up a magazine.

Jerry pulled the curtain, lathered Victor's groin area, and deftly removed his pubic hair.

"They'll start an IV soon, Mr. Newton." Jerry smiled and pattered out of the room.

Soon afterwards, Dr. Farrow came into the room, followed by Dr. Shum and a nurse.

"Mr. Newton, your biopsy results were as we expected." Dr. Farrow dragged the orange plastic chair to the side of the bed and sat down.

"Now, just to confirm, you have a carcinoma of the left lobe of the prostate. We will go ahead with surgery as planned tomorrow morning. Dr. Shum has pretty well explained everything; however, do you have any questions?" Dr. Farrow leaned back in the chair, folded his arms, and waited.

"I can't think of anything right now." Victor looked at me.

Dr. Farrow rose to his feet. "I'll see you in the morning, Mr. Newton. Mrs. Newton, may I have a word with you?" He motioned me out to the corridor.

"The surgery will begin at 8:00 a.m. There is no need for you to come to the hospital, Mrs. Newton, or to telephone. I will call you," he said. "That should be around noon if all goes well and we remove the prostate."

"Very well. Thank you, Doctor. Please be good to him," I added.

Dr. Shum walked quickly to catch up with the wiry Dr. Farrow as he entered the elevator.

～

"I'd like to meet this Doug Campbell before I have the surgery," Victor said thoughtfully.

"Let's go now before they bring that IV," I said, helping him into his housecoat. "We won't be gone too long."

The door to Doug Campbell's room was closed. We knocked and waited expectantly.

"Come in." The man in the bed pulled himself up with the aid of a bar handle attached to a chain secured to the ceiling, as we entered the room.

After we had introduced ourselves, Doug told us his story, not without some obvious bitterness.

"This should not have happened to me. I'm the last guy on earth this should happen to," he said angrily.

He was fifty-five, the manager of a hardware chain, living in the suburbs with his wife. He had two grown children. "I thought I had it all. I never smoked, I don't drink, and I'm a fitness buff. I've always been conscious of my diet and exercise program." Doug narrowed his eyes. "It didn't make a difference, did it?"

Victor could say nothing. I was anxious to talk about the operation.

"Are you able to get out of bed?" I asked.

"Oh sure, I'll be going home in another week. Let me tell you it's painful as hell, especially in the hips. I couldn't walk for a few days after the surgery. It's going to take time, but like

Dr. Farrow says, 'It's a cure.' He took out the whole damn prostate, but when you consider the alternative . . ." He shrugged
his shoulders.

Victor wished him luck. Doug asked Victor to close the door
on his way out.

It had stopped snowing and it was getting dark. From the
window on the second floor, we watched some of the staff
below scurrying home to dinner.

"Come on, angel, why don't you get something to eat."
Victor turned and led me to the elevator.

I didn't feel like eating, but I put in a half hour drinking
coffee so Victor wouldn't suspect and worry about me.

I attempted to leave several times after tucking him in and
arranging his things on the bedside table.

"Let's see, you have your water, tissues, pen and paper, and
Rob's number. I'll call as soon as I get to Rob's, okay, sweetheart?
I'll be here when you come out of the anaesthetic. I love you,"
I said, kissing his eyelids. I almost cried, but swallowed instead
and walked slowly out of the room.

Before I turned the corner onto University Avenue, I looked
back and saw him at the window throwing kisses until I was out
of sight.

~

Sleep would not come. After tossing and turning for hours, I
finally got up and looked at the clock. It was three o'clock in
the morning. Rob slept soundly as only a big healthy twenty-
five-year-old could.

I looked out of the window. It was snowing again.

I thought of my mother, impoverished, raising five children in a coal-mining town in Nova Scotia during the forties.

"Always remember," my mother would say, as she tucked me in at night. "When a storm passes through your life, it will make you stronger for the next one that is sure to follow. Now go to sleep and dream of glad tomorrows."

I awakened to the sound of the telephone ringing. Rob had already gone. I glanced at the clock and picked up the receiver. It was 9:10 in the morning.

"Mrs. Newton? Dr. Farrow here."

I was confused. "Dr. Farrow, you said you would call me at noon. Oh my God, is my husband dead?" I asked frantically.

"No, no, Mrs. Newton, now remember what I told you. If the cancer had spread, we would not remove the prostate. I'm sorry, but we found cancer cells in the surrounding lymph nodes."

My heart was pounding so loudly I could hardly hear him.

"He is in Recovery now," Dr. Farrow continued. "There's no point in coming down until he is back in his room, say about six this evening. We'll talk later, Mrs. Newton."

"Thank you, Doctor," I heard myself say in a voice I didn't recognize.

My mind was racing, trying to put it all together. It didn't matter what they told you to expect, it was hitting me fast and hard.

What did they say? Two to five years if the cancer had spread!

I fell to my knees on the mattress. All my pent-up rage and horror broke through in an explosion of gut-wrenching sobs and wails. When I could cry no more, I began to pray.

"Please, God. I can't bear it. Please help me," I implored. My body aching from grief, I fought for control as I made some tea and took a long, warm shower, breaking into wrenching sobs all over again.

I looked in the mirror at my swollen face. *Who do you think you are?* I scolded myself. *There are thousands in worse shape than you and Victor. What of the little children who are dying of leukaemia before their lives begin, like your brother Gerald? What would have become of you if Mom had fallen apart? She stayed strong for you and you have to stay strong for Victor. Now pull yourself together and take it an hour at a time until you can take it one day at a time. You're a Cape Bretoner. A survivor. Remember?*

~

Why am I so cold? Oh my God, I'm freezing. Where am I? Victor opened his eyes but he couldn't move. He wanted to call out, but he could only mouth the words.

Shivering uncontrollably, he looked to the left and saw a grey puffball head and another to the right, all lying on stretchers as he was. Some moaned and others moved slightly.

After what seemed like hours of freezing and shivering half to death – later he learned it was actually eight hours – a familiar face appeared and cheerily informed him that he was being taken back to his room.

"You'll feel better now, Mr. Newton," Jerry said, as he and a nurse completed the painful transfer from the stretcher to the bed.

"You can come in now, Mrs. Newton." Jerry checked the IV and the catheter. "He'll be out for a while yet."

Victor slipped in and out of a murky sleep. Finally his eyes began to focus. He became aware of soft lips on his brow and a warm hand holding his. "My angel," he whispered, "my Audrey," and he slipped away again.

When next he awoke his whole body was one huge terrible pain. Morphine dripped steadily from the IV into his veins, but it did not take away the pain fast enough. I wet his lips and gave him sips of ice water. He looked towards the window and asked me the time, noticing it was dark outside.

"It's six o'clock in the evening, Victor dear. You were in the recovery room all day. The nurse said you should have been back hours ago, but they had no one to bring you back. If I had known that earlier, I would have brought you back myself." I was churning with anger, but I did not want Victor to sense it. "Never mind, you're here now and that's what matters," I said.

"Have you seen Dr. Farrow?" he asked, eyes closed. "What did he do to me?"

"Victor dear, he did not remove your prostate," I replied, holding his hand expectantly.

Victor said nothing for a full minute and then to my surprise he said, "Good. I'm still a sexual man." He opened his eyes. "The thought of not being able to make love to my beautiful wife was harder to accept than any cancer. And besides," he added, "we're going to beat this." Closing his eyes, he drifted back into the fog, still holding my hand tightly.

~

The next few days were only half clear to him, half remembered, filled with horrible gas cramps and searing pain, IV poles, catheter bags, tubes, pills, and milky drink supplements.

"Mr. Newton, we want you to take this walker and walk as much as you are able." Jerry helped Victor to his feet.

Jerry was attentive and compassionate. He fashioned a loop and a steel bar rig so that Victor could pull himself up, as Doug Campbell had done when we had visited him, to lessen the strain on his stitches.

Victor positioned himself behind the walker and felt his knees turn to jelly. The support of the walker held him up and he made an effort to walk.

I made sure he did not overdo it the first time. The pain was excruciating but he pushed on. A few more steps and back to bed.

In less than a week he was doing laps around the corridors with a stubborn determination.

"All I want is to get the hell out of here," he said. Pushing the walker away, he walked to the end of the corridor and looked out of the window, turned around and walked back, steady and strong towards me.

~

Doug Campbell came with his wife, Pat, to say goodbye. He was going home. Smiling broadly, looking smart in his executive suit and topcoat, he shook Victor's hand and then suddenly dashed from the room, leaving behind a huge puddle of urine.

Doug's wife looked horrified. She glanced quickly around the room for something to clean it up.

"You go after him," I said. "He needs you now. I'll get some paper towels." I led Pat out of the room. I never saw them again.

I had been doing my homework, reading all I could get my hands on about the prostate, books from the library and articles in medical journals. Now I explained to Victor what had just happened to Doug.

"You see, Vitts, Doug had his prostate removed . . . a radical prostatectomy . . . one of the side effects of this surgery is loss of bladder control, especially noticeable when the catheter is removed. Sometimes incontinence can be a problem for months afterwards. Most men will have normal bladder function within a year. The patient is given exercises to do at home to strengthen the bladder, which is now attached directly to the urethra after the removal of the prostate gland."

"One more reason I'm glad I still have mine," Victor said, as he watched me wipe up the last drops of Doug's urine. "Poor devil."

~

The days turned into a week and Victor gained a little more strength. He was still in a lot of pain and he couldn't understand why. If they had not removed his prostate, why was he hurting so much? If the removal of the prostate was rough, what was it compared to the agony he was suffering now?

Victor asked Jerry if he could tell him anything more than Dr. Farrow had told him about the surgery.

"Did they cut my pelvic bone and pin it together again? Did they sit on me? Why was I black and blue from my waist to my knees?"

"You'll have to ask the doctor again." Jerry looked sympathetic. "It's an exploratory operation, Mr. Newton, and it can be painful, but I don't think they cut the pelvic bone." Jerry did remind him about the hormones he would have to take for the rest of his life, that would kill his sex drive.

"We'll see about that," Victor said, feisty as ever.

~

After the realization that he had cancer sank in, Victor experienced night terrors. He began to dream about caskets and cemeteries, waking up in a sweat.

My brother Joe came to see him. He had been with me the day after Victor's surgery. We were very close and Joe and Victor had become best friends.

Joe's a big friendly guy with a hearty laugh and a kind nature. Victor called him "good ole Joe," although he was twenty years his junior. Victor had taught him to paint and Joe had given up his job as security director for the Bay Centre to work full time at his art.

Victor's mind was at ease knowing I could count on Joe if I needed someone, especially if anything happened to him when he was in the operating room. *People die on operating tables every day. Why not me?* he had thought.

"Have you got everything?" I checked the locker and bedside table once more.

We stopped at the nurse's station and picked up the prescription for the hormone pills and pain medication and then walked towards the elevator. Victor never looked back.

When we were alone in the elevator he took me in his arms. "I want to kiss my wife. We're going home, sweetheart," he sighed. "We're going to see Cleo."

~

"Now look at that," I complained the next morning. "The plough just went by and blocked the driveway. I'll get the shovel, but you stay away from the door, Vitts. I don't want you to get a chill."

Victor handed me his big gloves. "Are you sure about driving to the vet's?" he asked. "I know how you hate driving."

"I have to, Vitts. Cleo and the cats will be going crazy, not to mention the boarding costs. I know you want to see them as much as I do," I said, closing the door and pushing the wide shovel down the long driveway towards the huge pile of snow.

Victor watched from the window in the family room while I struggled with the heavy snow. I had to stop periodically to lean on the shovel.

Although his appetite had not fully recovered, I prepared some of his favourite meals. Steak and mushrooms, baked potato and sour cream, green salad with blue cheese dressing, and strawberry cheesecake. He ate half-heartedly. He could no longer sit at the table because of the pain in his pelvis.

"I'm sorry, sweetheart, about your wonderful dinner, but if you don't mind I think I'll lie down." He shuffled slowly to the bedroom where I tucked him in and kissed his eyelids.

There was no improvement in Victor's condition in the days that followed. If anything, he was worse. After three weeks had passed, I called Dr. Farrow.

"Victor is having a lot of side effects from the hormone pills . . . diethylstilbestrol . . . his breasts are extremely painful and swollen, his belly is bloated, and the pain in his pelvis is very intense," I explained.

Dr. Farrow warned that the cancer would spread if Victor did not take the pills every day.

"He must stay on the diethylstilbestrol. The side effects will diminish as his body adjusts to the drug," Dr. Farrow said. "Let me see," he paused. "You have an appointment to see me on March 15. He should see some improvement by then."

Victor did not adjust. He could not and would not make peace with the dreaded hormone pills. His breasts became so painful that he could only describe it as if heavy pincers were hanging from each nipple. He wore his pyjamas and housecoat most of the time because he was in and out of bed all day and saw no point in getting dressed.

Each morning I brought him the two little pink hormone pills with his coffee. We both hated them now and would stare at the pills for a long minute before Victor swallowed them.

Victor cried often now, a side effect experienced by some patients after taking hormone therapy. We had both cried before, but now he was crying over the least little thing. Once he spilled his coffee when he bumped his elbow and he cried like a baby. If I became annoyed with him he cried inconsolably, great sobs shaking his body and the bed.

"For heaven's sake, Victor, you've got to pull yourself together," I scolded one morning. "You're not the only man in the world with prostate cancer. You can't stay in bed feeling sorry for yourself." I was shouting at him now, in tears myself.

He looked at me like a hurt little boy. Sobbing, he said, "I'm sorry, I don't know what to do."

My heart was breaking. "Oh God, Victor dear, I'm sorry too." I soothed and cradled him. "We're both under a great deal of stress."

"As long as you don't stop loving me," he said, searching my face.

"My love for you is boundless, endless." I looked deep into his eyes. "I don't want you to doubt that ever." I rested my head on his broad shoulder. "You know, Vitts, we're walking through a fire, but we're coming out. You'll see. So, what should we do today? How about a walk down the country road! We haven't been since we got the animals back. They'll love to walk with us again."

"I'm game," he said, getting out of bed with more determination than enthusiasm. He didn't mention the pelvic pain.

After the walk he brought two mugs of hot chocolate to the family room where I was reading my newest book, a guide to prescription drugs. "A new addition to your medical library I see," Victor said. He handed me the mug and let Cleo in for her afternoon visit.

The weeks passed slowly and painfully with no letup in the nausea, fatigue, and pelvic pain. Every morning I gave Victor the hated hormone pills. He no longer cringed at the sight of them. Instead, he swallowed them with sad resignation.

~

"I'm going to die," he said one morning, quite calmly.

I gripped him by the shoulders with a quiet fury. "No, you are not going to die," I said. "These goddamn pills are killing

you, not the cancer. Now listen to me, Victor, if you will coop-
erate and help me, you'll get better."

"Anything. I'll do anything you say because I believe in you,"
he said.

"All right, first of all I'm cutting the dosage of diethylstilbestrol in half. We have to taper off gradually. It's a powerful drug
and you can't stop taking it all at once or you may have serious
side effects. Next, you have to change your diet. I've been
telling you for years that you eat too much rich food. The more
I read about cancer, the more I realize what a significant role
fat plays in developing the disease. Starting tomorrow, no more
bacon and eggs. From now on it's going to be cereal, fruit, and
whole grain toast. No more steaks and cream sauces. We're
going to eat fish and lean chicken and lots of vegetables, tons
of broccoli. Okay?"

"Okay, boss," he replied, just as enthused. "Sounds good to me."

With the reduction in the hormones Victor began to feel
better. He was getting dressed and going for a walk down the
country road each day. His appetite improved and the side
effects slowly diminished, although he continued to experience
the pelvic pain and bloated belly. But he was well enough to
drive to Toronto for the appointment with Dr. Farrow on
March 15.

"Good to see you," the doctor said to Victor without making
eye contact with him. "How are you, Mrs. Newton?"

"We've cut the dosage of diethylstilbestrol in half," Victor
blurted out.

"I had intended to increase the dosage," Dr. Farrow said,
narrowing his eyes.

"I'm sorry, but I just can't take them. The side effects are killing me. I was getting worse instead of better." Victor was sounding defensive.

"Mr. Newton, this drug slows the production of testosterone, the male hormone that feeds the cancer. If you stop taking it the cancer will spread more rapidly. You must take it every day for the rest of your life," the doctor said.

"What about radiation?" Victor asked.

"Radiation. If you want radiation you can go to the Princess Margaret Hospital." The doctor was clearly indignant.

"I was just wondering," Victor said. "Is there anything else we can do?"

"We can do an orchiectomy, removal of the testicles. The testes produce the testosterone which acts on the cancer. It is a low-risk operation. The scrotum is opened, the testes are removed, and the skin is sewn up again. It is one of the oldest forms of treatment for prostate cancer." The doctor brought his fingertips together and waited for Victor's response. He received an unexpected one from me.

I stood up quickly. "Thank you, Doctor. We'll think about it. Let's go, sweetheart. We don't want to get caught in heavy traffic."

Victor was right behind me.

"I'll see you in six weeks," the doctor called after us. We did not reply.

~

Victor turned the car onto the highway and headed for home. "Now what do we do?" he asked, glancing at me, knowing I probably had something in mind.

63

"Let's stop at the shopping centre, Vitts. We'll have a cup of coffee and I can pick up that book I told you about. I was reading an article that indicated that it is the most comprehensive book you can read on cancer."

Later that evening Victor relaxed in the family room, with Cleo and the two cats curled up at his feet in front of the fireplace. I was reading the new book. It was pretty much up-to-date on almost every question you could think of.

"This book is amazing," I told Victor. "Just about everything you ever wanted to know about cancer but were afraid to ask."

Later, after looking through the book more thoroughly, I noted a list of cancer treatment centres in the back of the book. One of these centres was the Roswell Park Memorial Institute, which has a prostate cancer research and treatment centre in Buffalo, New York.

The following morning I was on the phone to Buffalo where a kind and patient lady listened to my story. She advised me to seek alternative treatment. "Take your husband to the Princess Margaret Hospital. You have one of the finest cancer treatment hospitals in the world in your backyard." She wished me good luck.

Because I needed a referral, I called Dr. Cronk in Belleville.

Dr. Cronk was distressed to learn that Victor had been sent to a surgeon in Toronto. "When I told your husband about radiation, Mrs. Newton, I fully expected he would be sent to the Princess Margaret Hospital. I'm very sorry. I'll call Dr. Ryder at the Princess Margaret Hospital now and they will be in touch with you."

I was smiling when I spoke to Victor. "I have a good feeling about this, Vitts."

"We'll know soon enough, sweetheart," he said. "Let's go for a walk before dinner. Come on, Cleo, it's a wonderful day. Let's go."

~

The next morning I awakened to the call of a phoebe. Victor had told me that according to folk wisdom, the small bird's call – two short notes followed by two more – means "Spring's here. Spring's here." It was April, and the temperature was rising and there was plenty of splishing, splashing rain. The weeks went by and the sun became stronger. The dreadful winter was over at last. Neighbours stopped by to offer a word of encouragement to Victor. They wished him well and presented him with jars of homemade jam, just-out-of-the-oven homemade bread, and luscious muffins. Someone left a bottle of dandelion wine.

An elderly couple who owned a small farm a few miles down the road came to visit. "Where there's life there's hope, Vic. Yer lookin' pretty good, boy," Frank said, patting Victor on the back. On their way out Maggie, known for her salty tongue, said, "Poor bastard, looks like hell. Don't he, Frank!"

It had been a rough winter. Victor had lost weight as well as colour. He had a naturally ruddy complexion that complemented his grey hair and green eyes. Now his skin was pale and dry and his cheeks hollow beneath dull eyes.

"It's going to be all right," I comforted him. "It's spring, Vitts. Everything is new again. We're going to the Princess Margaret

Hospital. I just know they are going to help you. You'll be on the golf course before you know it."

"You always make me feel good, sweetheart. I just hope they can tell me what's wrong with my pelvic bone." The pain and bloating had not diminished.

The bank continued to carry us, but the real estate people had failed to find a serious buyer. We lowered the price on the house for the second time. We had to face the hard facts. The bank would not carry us indefinitely. Something had to be done. What we needed was a miracle. In the meantime we lived as frugally as we could while coping with Victor's illness.

~

The postoperative pain and the effects of the hormone treatment, which drove us to seek an alternative radiation treatment, meant, finally that we found ourselves filling out forms again, this time at the Princess Margaret Hospital. We had heard about the famous hospital over the years and we knew people who had received treatment there. Some of what we had heard was positive, but we had also sensed the stigma of death due to cancer that was associated with it. Now we had to deal with our own fears and hopes, as we contemplated our first visit.

As we were leaving the parking lot and walking towards the hospital entrance, I stopped and took Victor by the hand. "Remember, Vitts. We're walking through the fire, but we're coming out. We've done it before, haven't we?"

"Right, sweetheart." He held the door for me and we walked into the Princess Margaret Hospital together.

What struck us immediately was the sense of order. There was no running and rushing about. Everyone smiled at us. The volunteers in their yellow smocks offered fresh coffee and cookies and sat down with the new patients to answer questions and generally talk about whatever the patient wanted to talk about. Most of the volunteers had lost someone to cancer. They knew the "cancer journey" well.

Victor and I sat facing another couple, a handsome well-dressed man in his late fifties with silver hair and a dark-haired, good-looking younger wife. They seemed very ill at ease and held each other's hands so tightly the whites of their knuckles showed.

I spoke first and soon there were introductions all around. The inevitable question was asked. "What brings you to the Princess Margaret Hospital?"

John, like Victor, had prostate cancer. John's doctor had sent him directly to the Princess Margaret Hospital, however, bypassing the exploratory surgery that Victor had endured.

Victor felt sympathy for John. Having had the hell scared out of him, he knew what John and his wife, Patti, were feeling. Although Patti seemed to resent the intrusion, John welcomed it and took in avidly all he could learn from Victor. Both men were called and sent to the laboratory to have samples of their blood taken. From there they were sent for chest X-rays. After that it was back to "Clinic J" to wait their turn to see the doctor.

Most of the various cancer clinics were open so that anyone walking by could see about twenty or thirty people sitting on black and chrome chairs watching one another, wondering what kind of cancer their fellow patients had as they waited to be called into the examining rooms. There were usually two urologists on duty in Clinic J at the same time. A patient was assigned to a physician and continued to see that same physician on each subsequent visit during the course of his or her treatment. John was called first, then Victor. In turn they disappeared behind the white door to be examined and digitally probed by the doctor, then given half a dozen requisition cards to take to the various departments of the hospital for the all-important tests that would determine the exact stage of their cancer and subsequent treatment.

Some of the tests were slated to be done in the following weeks, which meant we would be driving to and from the hospital over the course of the early summer.

~

Victor felt his anger welling up again whenever he thought about the hormone pills and the persistent pelvic pain.

"Dr. Ryder said those pills could cause me to have heart problems. You know, sweetheart, I'm still very angry, but at the same time I am absolutely elated with this hospital. I feel a true sense of caring here. It's as though a new door of hope has been opened up to me, to us," he added, patting my knee as he drove.

"We're coming through the fire, Vitts, but we still have a long way to go." We turned into our driveway and heard Cleo's welcome bark.

"Hey, Vitts. Come and see the sun going down behind George's cabin."

"That's not the sun going down, sweetheart, it's the moon coming up," he said, laughing.

"Well, it's the sunniest moon I've ever seen. My mother would have said it's a promise of better things to come and glad tomorrows. Let's have dinner, I'm starved," I said.

∼

The following week Victor was admitted to Princess Margaret Hospital for three days of intensive diagnostic testing including a biopsy of his prostate gland. As he placed his things on the bedside table, a familiar voice sounded behind him.

"Looks like we're roommates," John grinned, shaking Victor's hand. Patti busied herself unpacking John's things and I smiled with pleasure. I was happy to have the two men together again, knowing they would find comfort and support in one another.

It seemed to me that I could not imagine two more handsome, healthy-looking men. They both had beautiful grey hair. Victor had regained some of his natural high colour and John was tanned from hours of sunbathing at his cottage and winter skiing. They had strong features and were in good physical shape. They dressed smartly and had the demeanour of gentlemen. I felt a knot in my stomach as the reason for our being together in that room hit me. I felt the presence of the enemy – cancer – anxious to do battle, ready to take us on.

Well, the battle has begun, I thought, *and as in all battles there will be winners and losers. But by God, we will fight the good fight.*

Patti and I left the two men joking and laughing and headed for the city centre to do a little shopping. Neither man usually wore pyjamas, which prompted a lot of kidding, and so pyjamas were the first purchases we made.

~

Patti returned to her home in North Toronto each night, but I had to stay at the Princess Margaret Lodge. The lodge was a wonderful home away from home within sight of the hospital where the staff, volunteers, and out-patients all shared the common thread of dealing with an assortment of complex cancers.

It was usual to talk about one's own cancer. Patients and relatives gathered in the lounge in the evening, sipping cool drinks or hot tea and coffee made in the small kitchens located on each floor. They discussed their chemotherapy and radiation treatments. Without exception, each person would announce how many treatments were prescribed for them.

"Two down and twenty to go," volunteered a tall scrawny man in his sixties, whose lymphatic cancer had returned after a remission of fifteen years.

"Three more and I'll be finished," a middle-aged woman said, as she knitted at lightning speed, never taking her eyes off her audience.

Patients of various ages, a few as young as eighteen and some in their seventies, but mostly middle-aged women wearing an assortment of scarves and wigs to cover their balding heads, listened attentively to the newest member of the group tell her story.

Her name was Neena. She was thirty-two, the mother of two

small boys and a twelve-year-old girl. Her husband was caring for the children while she was taking treatment for ovarian cancer. Partway through her story she broke down and sobbed. "I'm so afraid for my children," she said. "I don't want to leave them. I don't want to die." She cried as two women, calming and comforting her, led her back to her room.

The men were different, not willing to show emotion. They either laughed and joked too much or remained silent, staring at television and magazines they did not see.

Victor awoke from the biopsy procedure in good spirits. Because this was his third biopsy, the previous two having been performed at Peterborough Civic Hospital and Toronto General, he had known what to expect. John, however, was not faring as well and found the minor surgery debilitating.

The day following the biopsy a nurse informed Victor that he was being released, and that Dr. Ryder would see him in his office with the results of this and previous diagnostic tests before he was discharged from the hospital.

"Come in, Mr. Newton. Oh, and ask your wife to come in also." Dr. Ryder was hunched over a mass of papers on his desk, glasses sitting on the end of his nose, Santa Claus-fashion.

"Do sit down, please. Now this is what we have found, Mr. Newton." Peering over his glasses, the doctor made eye contact with first Victor and then me. "You have a carcinoma, a tumour of both lobes of the prostate with the bulk of the disease in the left lobe; however, the cancer is contained within the prostate gland. Although the Toronto General found a few positive nodes, we have found no evidence of the cancer spreading in any other part of your body. No abdominal masses; bone scans are clear; liver function normal; chest X-ray clear; heart normal; kidneys normal. In other words, we could not do more if we went over you with a bacon slicer, Mr. Newton."

"That's wonderful," Victor said. "I'm grateful. But I still have cancer. What do I do now?"

"I'm sending you down to Planning on the first floor for a series of radiation treatments. They will mark you and tell you more about what to expect. You will probably get diarrhoea for a while and you will feel tired for a few weeks, but we hope to shrink the tumour and hold the cancer at bay. I'll see you here in the clinic from time to time and check on your progress." He got up from his chair. Taking Victor's extended hand, the doctor sandwiched it between both of his hands and said, "You know, Mr. Newton, they say if you are going to get cancer, prostate cancer is the one to get because it is slow-growing. But, I must caution you, some of these prostate cancers are very aggressive. We just don't know at this point."

"Thank you, Doctor. Thank you very much," Victor said. Dr. Ryder's frankness did not dampen his spirits in the least; in fact, he felt he was walking on air. He was all puffed up with hope. He felt now that he had a good fighting chance. Victor took me by the hand and walked with a spirited step towards the elevator. On the first floor, in Planning, he was given a new set of strategies and introduced to the newest weapon in his personal battle.

~

Victor began a course of twenty-one radiation treatments on July 9, 1982. Two permanent blue dots were tattooed on either side of his pelvis close to his hip bones to help guide the radiation to its mark, directly over the prostate. The treatments lasted only a few minutes and were given five days a week.

While sitting in the small waiting room in the basement of the hospital with people from all walks of life, we would suddenly be jolted out of the waiting-room lethargy by a mechanical-sounding voice broadcast over the PA system. Slowly, articulating each syllable, the voice would say, "Mr. New-ton to Linac. Mr. New-ton to Linac."

Victor would rise from his chair. All eyes would follow him until he disappeared from view. From the waiting room he walked down the hall to the heavy steel door marked "Linac," short for linear accelerator, the machine that delivered high-energy radiation to patients like Victor. This was where earlier he had deposited his appointment card – thereby confirming his arrival – in a box attached to the outside of the door. On a large sign in bold letters were the words "No Admittance: Medical Personnel Only."

One morning I saw John sitting in the laundry room. He looked tired and miserable. I asked him if he was all right and he explained that he did not want to be seen in case someone recognized him.

John had a law practice in the financial district and Patti thought it would be bad for business if his clients discovered that their lawyer had cancer. "I don't think I can take much more," John said. "I'm wiped out. Is Victor having any of this? How is he?"

"He's fine," I replied. I was puzzled. John looked terrible and yet he had been given the same number of radiation treatments as Victor. *My God!* I thought as I brought John a glass of water. *Maybe it hasn't hit Victor yet.* I couldn't understand it. Victor was playing golf after each treatment. "Is Patti here?" I asked.

"No, she's away for a few days visiting friends. Did you know she's an American? We've been married a year. All this cancer business is pretty hard on her. I sent her to Colorado for a week to visit her family," he said. He changed the subject. "I have a daughter. She wants to be a model." A tender smile came over John's face when he mentioned his daughter.

"Well, if she looks anything like her dad, she'll be a good one," I smiled back. "Would you like to join Victor and me for lunch?"

"No, no thank you, Audrey. Will you call a nurse for me?"

"Right away, John. You take care now. I'll see you later."

When Victor's treatment was over we looked for John, but we never saw him. I learned later that John had cancelled the rest of his treatments. We returned home feeling despondent.

"Twenty down, one to go, Vitts." I checked the appointment card again. "How are you feeling today?" He was a little more pale than usual.

"Except for the diarrhoea and fatigue, not too bad," he replied as he steered the car onto the highway and headed towards Toronto for his final radiation treatment.

"You know how very grateful I am, sweetheart. A few months ago I thought I was going to die. Now I don't think like that any more."

~

"Now Mr. Newton, I'll see you in six weeks," Dr. Ryder said. "You go home and carry on as you normally would. Your energy will return slowly but you'll get it back." He slapped Victor gently on the back as he led him to the door. He cut short our effusions of gratitude.

Driving home we were jubilant.

"Sing one of your Cape Breton songs for me, sweetheart. In fact, you can sing all of them." I sang all the way home.

"I think I'll lie down before dinner. I feel exhausted." Victor undressed and lay on the bed. "Will you put your healing hands on my stomach?" he asked. "It's pretty sore."

"I'll massage it with a little lotion." I was about to begin when I yelped, "What's this?"

"What? What is it?" Victor strained to look at his belly.

"Don't tell me you know nothing about it!" I handed him a mirror and when he held it over his belly, a big round smile face was grinning back at him. "Those little devils. The X-ray technicians did that. They knew it was my last treatment," he laughed.

"What were you doing behind those doors?" I chided. I knew all too well that Victor could inject a little fun and humour into the most serious situations. I once said he could make a prune smile. Later I was sorry I had not taken a picture of the smile face below his belly button.

"Guess what," Victor grinned smugly.

"What?" I reached for the towel and dried my hands. "This had better be good. I'm in the middle of making fish cakes."

"I felt a stirring down there this morning. I think it's coming back."

"That's wonderful, sweetheart. I told you it would after Dr. Ryder took you off the diethylstilbestrol. So, what do you think?" I was teasing him.

"I think," he said reaching for me, "that I will think about it . . . all day long." He kissed my neck, my shoulder, all the way down my arm to my fingertips.

"You think about it," I laughed. "I've got fish cakes to make."

After dinner he placed the big duvet and pillows on the floor in front of the fireplace along with a bottle of white wine. He lowered the music and waited. Trying not to feel anxious, he heard my soft steps and turned to see me standing in the doorway. I was wearing the long pink woolen scarf and tuque he had given me one Christmas.

"My angel, you take my breath away," he said as he welcomed me to his waiting arms.

The following day while on our usual walk down the country road he stopped, took me in his arms, and said, "Thank you for not giving up on me. I've never been happier. You can't imagine how I feel. I'm a man again."

"I never doubted it for a minute," I said. "Come on, I'll race you this time," I laughed, and we ran all the way home with Cleo and the cats in glad pursuit.

~

"You're taking the radiotherapy very well, Mr. Newton. I'm not too surprised you had an erection. Good for you." Dr. Ryder sounded like a school teacher praising his favourite pupil. "Radiation therapy is highly misunderstood," he continued. "In some cases it's true there is a loss of libido, but there are usually other complications that contribute to impotence. Sometimes it's psychological. Just because the patient is receiving radiation, he believes his sex life is over and doesn't bother any more. As we can see, Mr. Newton, that is not necessarily so." Dr. Ryder looked at the file again. "I'll see you in three months." He stood up and shook Victor's hand vigorously. "Goodbye, Mr. Newton. You're doing well."

~

It was late fall. We had not yet sold the house. Victor and I were very anxious and so was the bank. It could not carry us much longer. The twenty-five-thousand-dollar loan was reaching maturity and would not be extended.

"We'll just have to apply for some kind of assistance, Vitts, until we sell the house," I said as I looked up the address of the social assistance offices.

"Whatever you say. I don't have the strength to argue." His belly bloated and painful, Victor remained in the car as I walked into the office of Peterborough Social Services.

"I'm sorry, Mrs. Newton. We cannot be of assistance to you because you own a house. You don't qualify."

"But we've had the house for sale for almost a year now and we've lowered the price from $150,000 to $75,000. The bank will take it. I don't know what to do." I was in tears. "My husband is sick, battling cancer."

The man with the kind eyes looked at me thoughtfully. "Tell me, Mrs. Newton, has your husband been in the armed services?"

By coincidence the night before I had been looking at

Victor's Bible, left to him by his father, and had come across his army discharge papers.

For a moment I did not know if this information would go with or against us and I answered hesitantly.

"Well, I think he was in the army for a few years, but that was a long time ago."

"That's wonderful," he said, rising from his chair.

"It is?" I said puzzled.

"Where is your husband, Mrs. Newton?"

"He's waiting for me in the car. He didn't feel well enough to come in."

The counsellor came with me to talk with Victor.

"Mr. Newton," he said, "you don't qualify for social assistance, but I think you will qualify for one of the best pensions in this country, a War Veteran's Pension. The office is just down the street over the post office. They will look after you."

Knowing how this was embarrassing him, I volunteered to see the people at the Department of Veteran Affairs (as it was then called) myself. When I returned to the car Victor could see that I was smiling broadly and his heart rose. "You qualify, Vitts," I said, kissing him quickly. "All we have to do is fill out the forms and send in your discharge papers from the army and you will receive a monthly pension."

Victor's eyes filled with tears. "God has truly looked after us," he said. "What made you look in the old Bible?"

"I don't know. An angel, I guess."

"I have a brilliant idea, sweetheart."

"You're full of brilliant ideas," I said. "What is it this time?" I brought coffee into the family room and placed another log on the fire. Victor told me of his plan.

Using a good photo of our house, Victor created his own listing and had two dozen copies made. I jumped out of the car to drop a copy into every real estate office within a forty-mile radius with an offer of 6 per cent commission to the salesperson who would bring us a buyer. In less than two weeks we had sold the house for seventy-five thousand dollars. We signed an early closing and made a deal with the new owners to pay rent until we found a place to live.

However, we decided to vacate as soon as possible even though Victor was feeling the cumulative effects of the radiation, along with the pelvic pain from the original surgery, which had not yet subsided. He was in constant pain and distress. His stomach was so bloated he could not do up his pants even after I had let them out a few inches. We decided to move to Peterborough.

Now we had to part with Cleo, Pierre, and Bebe. I found a home for Cleo with a farm family and we placed the cats with the Humane Society to be adopted. The animals were very frightened and a lot of tears were shed when we said goodbye.

The following day we sold a truckload of our furniture to an auction house and put the rest in storage. Then we checked into a motel outside of Peterborough and fell exhausted into bed. The next day we met with our lawyer for a final reckoning. After the sale of the house and the repayment of the bank loan, the balance coming to us was twelve thousand dollars.

Victor felt more discouraged than ever and blamed himself for everything. I reminded him that we had lived very well on his investments for more than seven years.

"Don't worry," I told him. "We're going to be okay. We'll find a place of our own and begin a new life. It'll be an adventure. We have each other, Vitts, and that's all that really matters. Remember our wonderful wilderness canoe trips? All we had was a tent, and you said if we were ever lost in the woods we would survive as long as we had each other. We're a little lost now, but we will survive."

"Come here," he said, reaching for me. "Any other man might have committed suicide," he said, holding me close.

"Not you, Vitts." Tears trickled down my cheeks. "Not you. You're a survivor. Come on, let's get some sleep. Tomorrow we look at houses."

The real estate agent had several houses to show us. The first one was priced at thirty-five thousand. It was a three-storey house. Because it was the least expensive, we decided to negotiate a deal.

Back at his office, the agent continued to jot down figures and percentages. "I have to be frank with you," he said. "I don't think you will be able to get a mortgage with ten thousand down with no income other than your pension.

"If you can come up with another ten thousand dollars there would be no problem. That would leave you with a mortgage of fifteen thousand, probably at 15 per cent. The rates are high right now."

Victor's shoulders sagged and my face dropped as we left the real estate office and returned to the motel. Victor was ill, depressed, and in pain. I tried to get him to eat something but he would only drink coffee. "It's going to be okay, Vitts," I tried to comfort him. "We'll find something," I said, my voice betraying my faked confidence.

To cut down on expenses, we were eating one meal a day at the cafeteria in Eaton's. I made sure Victor was getting enough nourishment, buying oranges and milk for breakfast and cheese for snacks. It was in the Eaton's cafeteria when we were about to have a hot meal that Victor began to experience chest pain and an irregular heartbeat. I ushered him out immediately and took him to Emergency at the Civic Hospital where he was diagnosed with premature ventricular contractions, a frightening, irregular heartbeat. He was stabilized and released.

"It's all too much stress, sweetheart," I said, as I tucked him into bed. To make matters worse, the septic tank on the motel property was leaking and the stench was unbearable. Because Victor was still nauseous from the radiation, we had to move to another motel a mile down the road. Victor stayed in bed more often than not for the next few days.

I remembered a girlfriend who was working in real estate in Peterborough. I gave her a call and related our plight to her. "I don't believe this," Lee said. "I have the perfect house for you. My friend, Mary, told me this morning she wants to sell her house on Chamberlain Street. I was just about to list it. Meet me at 590 Chamberlain Street this evening at 8:00 p.m. and I'll show it to you."

When I told Victor about Lee and the house, he said, "You will have to go, sweetheart. I'm too sick. You can take a taxi. It should only cost about five dollars, but I think you are wasting your time. We don't have the money."

I returned a few hours later, excited and anxious. "Victor, you will love this house. It's a hundred times better than the one we looked at last week. It's a beautiful old house, two and a half storeys with two huge blue spruce trees in front and a big back-yard with grapevines. Wait till you hear this, Vitts: it has a wine cellar. An Italian family owned it at one time."

"Did he leave any wine?" Victor joked. He became interested as I described the house.

"There would be plenty of room for an art studio and it even has a wood stove. I know you, Vitts, and I just know you will love it."

"I don't want to dampen your spirits, but we still need another ten thousand dollars. How much is this house?" he asked, expecting it to be much more than the one we had looked at.

"The same price," I said excitedly. "Can you believe it? Thirty-five thousand. I've thought of something you may not agree to, but it's our only chance, Vitts." I sat on the bed, legs tucked beneath me, and took a deep breath.

"Let's hear it," he said, not opening his eyes.

"I'll go to Toronto on the bus and ask ten of your closest friends, those who we know are well off, to loan us one thou-sand dollars each. You see, it is much easier to loan one thou-sand than it is to loan ten thousand and it would be much easier for us to pay back one thousand at a time. I'm sure they will all want to help; they are lifelong friends. They would be hurt if you didn't ask. They were guests at your cottage and golf stags for years. They'll want to help. That's what friends are for."

"Well, okay, sweetheart, if you have that kind of faith, I'm with you all the way. It seems you are fighting all my battles these days."

I smiled at him. "Go to sleep, darling. Everything will be all right." I snuggled against him, felt his warmth, and listened to his deep breathing mingled with the patter of a November sleet against the frail window-panes of the motel.

Armed with a list of ten of Victor's closest, dearest, and most prosperous friends, I stepped off the bus and braced myself against the biting sleet and rain as I made my way into the street. I decided to make the calls away from the busy bus terminal and I found a telephone booth half a block away. I poured out my tearful story first to Tim, a friend Victor had gone skiing with the year before, along with another friend, Gord. Both men had executive positions in their professions. I held my breath as I heard Tim say, "Well, Audrey, I don't know. I . . . uh . . . well, you just don't lend that kind of money."

"It's only a thousand," I pleaded.

"Look, you people had better forget about a house and rent instead." He sounded irritated. I apologized for bothering him. I dialled Gord's number. Gord, who had a mild stammer, was stammering uncomfortably now. "You see, Audrey, I'm having personal problems at home, and I don't know where that will leave me financially." Again I said I was sorry to have bothered him.

I stepped out into the rain and took a deep breath. I thought of Victor back at the motel, his belly swollen with pain and nausea, his spirit broken, and my tears fell with the rain as I walked the street not knowing what to do or where to turn. I knew Victor did not want me to, but I decided to call his family. It was my last hope. I telephoned his sister Anne's number and got his niece, Molly. I asked if they would help. Molly hesitated.

"Give me your number," she said. "I'll have to think about it and call you back in about ten minutes."

I waited, shivering in the cold booth, and jumped when the phone rang. "I talked to Mom," Molly said. "Give me an address. She is going to send eight thousand dollars and Chuck is sending the other two, okay?" Molly was anxious to end the call.

Overcome with emotion, I could hardly speak. I thanked Molly and fell to my knees in the telephone booth and sobbed with relief.

In the washroom back at the bus terminal, I washed my face and put on lipstick. I had only minutes to catch the evening bus back to Peterborough. I had not been away from Victor for any length of time since the onset of his illness and now I was anxious and worried.

The coach sped along the highway through the rain as I thought about the calls I had made to Victor's friends. I decided not to tell him about them. I was angry, but most of all saddened by their lack of compassion.

Victor lay on the bed exactly as I had left him. I tried to sound excited when I gave him my news, but I was exhausted. "Your sister Anne and your brother Chuck are sending the cheque tomorrow. Isn't it wonderful, Vitts? We're getting the house. Oh, I must call Lee and tell her right away. Are you listening?" Victor hadn't opened his eyes and now I saw the tears on his cheeks. I leaned over and kissed them. He reached out and put his arms around me.

"Ah, come on Vitts, cheer up. We still have a bottle of Chablis. I've been saving it for something special and this is the moment." When I had poured the wine, I clicked my glass against his. "Here's to our new life on Chamberlain Street. Everything is going to be all right. I just know it is."

Later as we lay in the darkness side by side he said, "You called them, didn't you? Tell me, I can take it." So I told him. "I'm not surprised," he sighed. "I haven't heard from any of them since I lost the money and got cancer."

"Well, I am." I was angry again. "How could they do that to you? These are friends you have known for more than thirty years! How could they be so insensitive? How could they not care?"

"I have nothing to offer them any more," Victor said. "Let's forget it, sweetheart. You need to get some sleep. I have you and that's all that matters." He fell asleep with his arm firmly linked with mine.

One Day at a Time

Cancer alters lives. For those men whose prostate cancer is detected in Stage A who are appropriately treated, a complete cure may result. Similarly, cases of prostate cancer found in Stage B, while more unpredictable, are also frequently cured. For the men who are cured, the effect of cancer may be only a more acute sense of the fragility and impermanence of their lives. For a fortunate few, the experience may even be stimulating, encouraging a new, more intense approach to daily living. But for those whose prostate cancer can only be treated, not cured, the consequences are different.

There is no cure for prostate cancer that has metastasized beyond the prostate gland itself. With proper treatment and, perhaps, a modicum of good luck, the patient's life may yet be relatively long, vigorous, and useful. Victor lived for more than ten years after he was diagnosed with a Stage D1 cancer in his lymphatic system. Up until the final few months, he remained physically active and mentally alert. In fact, he lived a good deal longer than he was initially expected to live. I believe that his example should inspire hope in others, not only because he lived so long after the disease was discovered, but also, and especially, because he continued to get so much out of life.

Some of the adjustments the patient must make are, obviously, physical; others are psychological, affecting the way he thinks about himself and how he gets along with others. The significant people in his life have to make adjustments, too, as the patient's role is altered. The following notes reflect my experience and Victor's when, together, we learned to live with prostate cancer.

What the Patient Goes Through
Pain and Discomfort

The most obvious and continuing effects of prostate cancer are physical. Both the disease itself and the side effects of the treatments are a continuing concern to the patient and a preoccupation of the doctors who do their best to alleviate them. Unfortunately, there are limits to what the medical profession can do. Not all questions are answerable; not all problems can be solved. In Victor's case, the exploratory surgery he underwent in the first year of his battle with the disease had long-lasting effects. The source of his difficulties was never satisfactorily revealed – it was simply a rough procedure – and only time gradually made him better.

Of course, any symptoms, side effects, and aftereffects should be reported to the doctor. And a second opinion should always be made available if the patient is dissatisfied. And bear in mind that the patient needs the moral support of his spouse or supporter to get the answers to which he is entitled.

Altered Circumstances

Prostate cancer and some of the treatments that are prescribed for those who have it can be debilitating. In addition to the specific side effects of surgery, radiation, and hormone therapy, for example, the patient is likely to be fatigued. He may not be able to do things that he used to be able to do easily. For an active man, the loss of strength and stamina can be especially hard to take.

The fact that this disease, in particular, attacks a man at the source of his masculinity, sometimes robbing him of sexual potency, is another factor contributing to his feeling of vulnerability and unaccustomed weakness.

The physical decline often has practical consequences: the patient with prostate cancer, if he is not already retired, may lose time from work or be unable to continue working. The loss of income may mean that he has to make other changes in his way of life. For the individual who has long seen himself in the role of breadwinner, the change may lead to a loss of confidence and self-esteem. Many men, finding themselves in this situation, become depressed.

The psychological effects of disease can be treated no less effectively than the physical effects. But first they must be recognized and acknowledged. Both the patient and the people who are close to him should watch for signs of depression and seek the advice of health professionals in dealing with them.

Loss of Control

Closely tied to the physical and (sometimes) psychological effects of the disease in cases where it is progressing is the patient's increased dependence on others. Doctors and other medical professionals suddenly play a large role in his life, making important decisions affecting his comfort and, indeed, his continued survival. Similarly, the patient is likely to depend more heavily on the advice and love and affection of the people closest to him. These adjustments in relationships can be difficult for everyone.

Fear of Death

When a man is diagnosed with prostate cancer, the first thing he may think is that he is going to die. Perhaps, as an older man – prostate cancer is rarely found in men under the age of fifty, and is often found in men in their sixties and seventies – he may have been wrestling already with thoughts of his mortality, thoughts now intensified by the diagnosis. He is likely to feel a number of mixed emotions, ranging from fear and anger, to sadness and depression.

There is no cure for mortality, of course, nor for the fear it engenders. We each face the end in our own way. But any disease, including prostate cancer, may be easier to accept and deal with if the patient knows what he is up against. And it can also be helpful to share feelings with others. At the time Victor battled the disease, men often found themselves psychologically on their own: most men didn't want to admit that they had prostate cancer. This situation is changing rapidly. Today, there are support groups springing up all over the country where men can find the latest information about the disease and the advice and shared experiences of other patients. See the back of the book for more information.

Altered Relationships

A number of surprising things happened to Victor when news of his cancer was heard by others. A few long-time friends stopped calling. Victor was hurt at first but he came to understand that these people were afraid they would say the wrong thing. He soon put them at ease by talking about his prostate cancer readily and openly.

Other "friends" dropped him. Some, I think, were simply afraid of cancer. Others, as Victor himself observed, decided that he had nothing left to offer them. This happens.

Men with prostate cancer may discover, either with joy or sadness, the depth and sincerity of their relationships with other people. Some men we encountered in the course of our experience with the disease seemed to be profoundly alone.

What the Caregiver Must Do

The person who finds herself or himself caring for a man with prostate cancer should be aware, first of all, of what he is going through. The caregiver's essential role is to respond positively to the patient's needs.

The caregiver may have to make decisions for the patient that, in previous times, he would have made himself. He or she will have to help the patient come to terms with the disease. In the majority of situations, of course, the patient will have established a solid relationship with his doctor. And the doctor, in turn, will be making appropriate decisions with respect to treatment. Still, there may be a continuing role for the caregiver or supporter. This may mean sitting in on the patient's meetings with doctors, asking questions, learning about the disease, and understanding the options available.

Sometimes, the caregiver's role is to be alert to changes in the patient's condition. When prostate cancer has metastasized to other parts of the body, for example, new, and sometimes alarming, symptoms may occur. The one who is closest to the patient may notice these changes before the doctor does. They should be reported to the doctor as soon as possible, so that appropriate measures can be put into effect. Examinations and tests will indicate what further treatment will be given.

Above all, what the patient needs most from the caregiver is to feel that he is not alone.

Doctors

Most doctors are dedicated and competent. Some are selfless and gifted to an astonishing degree. Anyone who has an illness that requires treatment over a long period of time is likely to encounter all kinds of doctors. And just about everyone in this situation is likely to form a high regard for the profession as a whole.

Occasionally, doctors may be mistaken. Patients are entitled to expect that any course of action is fully explained. Most doctors nowadays accept this as a matter of routine. When recommending a procedure or drug therapy, they should describe the risks and alternatives clearly. Make sure they do even if it requires a degree of courteous persistence on your part, either as patient or caregiver. And have faith in your own instincts. We found more than once, Victor and I, that we were justified in getting another opinion when we weren't satisfied with the first one offered.

Unconventional Treatments

If the prostate cancer patient's condition becomes terminal, he may be tempted to seek alternative and controversial treatments. This is understandable. When an individual is presented with the grim news that his condition is terminal, it is not surprising that he would want to investigate alternative treatments that seem to offer hope. No doubt he will have heard about amazing cancer "cures," as most of us have, through the media or well-meaning friends. However, the patient should be very cautious and find out about the legal, moral, and financial costs of embarking on an unconventional and unproved treatment for cancer. Some individuals have wasted enormous sums of money in the pursuit of a non-existent remedy. They have sacrificed time and hope, too, that might have been expended more realistically.

There is, in addition, some danger involved in taking a new substance along with traditional treatment, which could cause physical distress. I would strongly advise anyone who is considering this course to speak with your doctor first, and discuss your feelings with your family, so that they are aware of your intentions.

The Princess Margaret Hospital

For both Victor and me the Princess Margaret Hospital in Toronto came to be a special place. We found the doctors there to be particularly committed, caring, and knowledgeable. We looked upon it as a lifeline, eagerly grasped when we were in despair, and I can honestly say that the doctors there never let us down.

It is not the only such hospital in Canada. Nor are the doctors there unique. Perhaps all prostate cancer patients find their own version of the Princess Margaret Hospital, in that they accept treatment for the disease and put their trust in a particular doctor or institution as part of the process of learning to live with it.

In any event, it would be a mistake to think, just because our experience there was so positive, that only the Princess Margaret Hospital provides first-class care for cancer patients. Expert care is widely available. The patient's task (assisted by those closest to him) is to make sure that he finds it.

Victor and I moved into the big red brick house on Chamberlain Street on the first day of December 1982. We had $150 left over after making the down payment and paying the legal and moving expenses. We still had Victor's pension coming in, but after the mortgage, utilities, and insurance were paid, we would have about $130 a month for food, heat, and living expenses. I thought about going back to work, and we discussed the possibility, but Victor wanted me with him. He needed looking after. He still had not recovered from the surgery.

"You know, sweetheart, when you told me about this house you didn't tell me we would be living in a factory town. Come and look." Victor pointed to a group of old brick buildings visible from the window of his art studio on the second floor of the house. The window looked north: every art studio should have north light, he had told me. It's the purest light to paint by.

"Oh, I forgot to tell you. It's the Canadian General Electric Plant. It's huge, a whole city block. Maybe they'll buy a few paintings." I craned my neck for a better view. The window also looked over the backyard and the tall maple and chestnut trees towering over the grapevine trellises now covered with snow. With his artist's eye, Victor had no trouble imagining the lush beauty of the yard in summer. *Audrey will love it*, he thought as he unpacked his art supplies.

Suddenly he was gripped by pain and nausea. He made his way slowly to the bedroom and then stopped and looked in the full-length mirror at his swollen abdomen. "Looks like a bloody watermelon. What the hell can I do? It's been almost a year."

"We can go back to the Princess Margaret Hospital," I said. He lay on the bed and I massaged his belly with a cooling lotion as I had many times before.

"I asked Dr. Ryder if Dr. Farrow cut my pelvic bone. He said he didn't know." Victor groaned.

"Well, it's not side effects from the radiation causing the pelvic pain because you had pain before the radiation." I continued massaging. "There has to be an explanation. I can't find anything in *The Merck Manual* to explain it."

Victor was angry. "I'm going to write to Dr. Farrow and ask him to tell me exactly what he did to me during that surgery. This pain is tormenting me and I want some answers. Getting the house and the pension were wonderful breaks, but what good are they if my life is rat shit? And yours, too, sweetheart."

"We'll find out, Vitts. Don't worry, we'll find out." I lay down beside him and kissed his eyelids.

~

Christmas came, but again there wasn't any money. The girls went to their mother's. Victor and I both felt the weight of the day and were glad when it was over. We did, however, accept an invitation to a holiday party in Toronto from Sue and Tom, dear old friends of Victor. We looked forward to seeing people we had not seen for more than a year and to a change of scene. I was thrilled to be getting into some party clothes and Victor whistled while he showered. Tom and Sue greeted us warmly.

"It's good to see you all again," Victor said making his way towards a group of men, shaking hands and smiling warmly.

"So you're all right now, eh?" Bob said, backing away from Victor. I looked across the room and met Tim's eyes. Embarrassed, he looked away quickly, no doubt remembering the telephone call and my desperate plea for help. I held out my hand to Gord and he stammered uncomfortably. It occurred to me that it may have been a mistake to have come. And then, suddenly I felt a hand grip my shoulder and I was spun around by Gord's wife, Lizzie.

"How dare you call Gord, begging for money!" She was yelling at me and attracting the attention of everyone in the room.

"I'm sorry," I said, alarmed. "I didn't mean to offend anyone. Victor was very ill and we were looking for help."

"I don't want to hear your sick stories, you selfish creature!" Lizzie said, and stalked away in a huff. Victor suggested we leave.

In the week following the party we received calls from about half the people who had witnessed Lizzie's outburst. They conveyed their sympathy and support for Victor and me, and distress at the scene they had witnessed.

~

One evening Victor took me by the hand and led me to the living room window. "Look at the beautiful lights," he said with his arms around me. It was dark outside and a soft snow was falling, melting as it hit the pavement.

"When I was a child in Glace Bay we always got barley sugar candy in our Christmas stockings," I said. "They looked like small stained glass animals, in red, yellow, and green. The stoplights at the intersection reflecting on the wet pavement remind me of my Christmas candy."

"You're still a little girl sometimes," Victor said, as he imagined the barley sugar animals dancing on the wet pavement.

It had been a month since we had given away Cleo. She had been adopted by a farm family near Hastings. I telephoned the family one day to find out how she was adjusting to her new home and was devastated to learn that she had run away. She had already been gone three weeks. It was no use asking why we had not been informed and there was little point in reproaching them. Victor advertised on the radio and placed a description of Cleo in all the local newspapers. We drove for miles along the country roads around her last home, searching and calling her name, but it was no use: there was too much territory to cover. And then, on New Year's Day, we received a call from a lady near the town of Campbellford. A big black dog had been living under her trailer for two weeks.

"We're on our way," I said, and in less than an hour we were reunited with our beloved Cleo. She had lost weight but was in pretty good shape considering the ordeal she had been through. The lady's son had given her table scraps every day. Cleo jumped into the back seat of the car and swished her tail all the way to our new home.

"How do you think she will take to city life, Vitts? The country is all she has ever known."

"Sweetheart, that dog will be happy wherever you are. She'll be just fine," he said. He patted my knee. "We adjusted, didn't we?"

~

The continuing discomfort in Victor's abdomen was a source of unending aggravation. He blamed Dr. Farrow for it: he was convinced that the surgery had been mishandled. Looking back on it now from a calmer perspective, this seems unlikely. Surgery, as Dr. Farrow himself had agreed, can be rough on the patient. Victor was hurting, but he did, gradually, recover from the effects of the procedure.

I wonder now if the anger Victor directed at Dr. Farrow was actually part of a larger anger about what had happened to him. Victor was a thoughtful, intelligent and rational man. He understood – we both understood – that cancer is something that just happens. But maybe in the part of us that doesn't think, but feels, we felt the need to blame someone for the disease that we knew would end Victor's life.

In any event, when Victor received no reply to his first letter to Dr. Farrow he wrote another, stronger one. The answer came in less than a week. "Listen to this." Victor read the letter aloud to me.

In the letter, which was brief and to the point, Dr. Farrow wrote that he had no recollection of having received Victor's first letter. He went on to describe the surgery in which, he indicated, five lymph nodes had been biopsied, and one found to be malignant. No other malignancy was found and no evidence of nerve damage was discovered. That was all.

"I distinctly asked him why I continue to have pain in the pelvis and why I was black and blue from my waist to my knees after he operated on me and he has not answered those questions," Victor complained.

"He says there was no evidence of cancer elsewhere, except one node," I said, studying the letter. "Vitts, we just have to conclude that it was a rough operation and that it will take a long time to recover."

"I think I'll lie down." Victor was clearly agitated and disappointed. "I'm sorry, sweetheart; this must be awful for you."

"Don't be sorry, Vitts. I'm with you all the way. We're going to beat this together." I kissed him. "Who loves who around here anyway?"

~

By the summer of 1983 Victor was feeling better, even playing golf a few times a week. He assessed the pain in his pelvis for me on a scale of one to ten: "I would say about a four, but it's still there. I get used to it when I'm busy. It bothers me mostly at night," he said. The bloating in his belly had gone down considerably but now something else was niggling at his comfort. He noticed blood with every bowel movement. He said nothing to me until he passed an alarming amount of blood one morning and asked me to look at it.

"I'll call the doctor here in Peterborough, Vitts. It may be haemorrhoids. They can bleed quite profusely at times. Don't worry, we'll find out what it is."

"I'm not worried," he said, "unless it ruins my golf game!"

"You see, Mr. Newton, this bleeding is to be expected as a side effect of the radiation," the youthful but self-assured doctor explained. He looked as though he had just stepped out of medical school. "You will no doubt experience it from time to time. Let me know if you have any other problems." He showed us to the door.

The following week I called him again.

"I'm really worried, Doctor. Victor is passing blood every day. He is getting weak."

"Now, Mrs. Newton, it looks like a lot, I know, but you mustn't worry so much. You guys should get on with your life. Perhaps I could prescribe something for your anxiety."

"Before you do that I'm sure you won't mind if I get another opinion," I said, and hung up.

Later that same evening I called Patti to find out if John was having any problems. Patti told me that John had died of his prostate cancer the previous March. Victor was devastated by the news.

~

The bleeding stopped. Victor resumed his golf and painting while I marketed his work. I wrote profiles and brochures and had them printed. I sent out business cards and placed advertisements in the local newspapers. A few local papers published articles about him. They described him as an important addition to the local art scene and invited the public to view his "wonderful realistic landscapes" of the Kawartha Lakes and woods at the gallery in our home on Chamberlain Street.

"Hi, Vitts." I peeked into the art room.

"Where have you been? You were going to bring me a cup of tea," Victor said, not taking his eyes off the painting he was working on as he stroked his brush across the canvas. A stark tree emerged against a soft, cloudy, peach-coloured sky.

"I was in the C.G.E. plant. I sneaked out with one of your paintings. I wanted to surprise you." I was breathless now and beamed at him.

"Wait till I clean my brushes. I'll come down and have that tea with you and you can tell me all about it."

When he joined me, I told him my news. "I suggested the company include an original oil painting as a gift along with the traditional watch and camera for their forty-year service award recipients. They thought it was a great idea. Now you are on the list and all we have to do is wait for our first customer. They choose a painting, we get a plaque made with their name on it, and then deliver the painting to the office with our bill and wait for the cheque!"

"That's wonderful," he said. "I want a kiss." He hugged and kissed me and told me how proud he was of me. "I'll have to get busy," he said looking around the room. We'll need a few more frames."

"Every time we sell a painting we'll invest in more frames until we have the walls covered. Every wall," I said. "Someday we won't find space to hang another painting because you will have painted so many; there just won't be room. I know you, Vitts. You can and you will do it."

"You're something else," he said. He was laughing as he headed upstairs to the art room.

By summer's end we had sold five paintings and had made enough money to buy two dozen frames. We also had enough money to buy a new airtight stove with a glass door so we could see the fire on long winter evenings.

All seemed well until the bleeding started again. We had changed doctors but we were again reassured that the bleeding was caused by radiation colitis, or inflammation of the lining of the colon. The bleeding persisted. I called Dr. Ryder who told me that it was probably caused by radiation, which could produce a kind of shredding effect on the bowel, causing it to bleed. I asked him why we had not been told to expect it at the beginning of the therapy. He explained that it occurs in only about 5 per cent of patients and they did not want to upset the other 95 per cent. Victor continued to bleed intermittently in the weeks that followed. He was still bleeding in December and there was no indication that it would subside. I called Dr. Ryder at the Princess Margaret Hospital again.

"What did he say?" Victor asked apprehensively.

"He seems to think I'm in a panic," I replied.

"Well, sweetheart, they are the experts," Victor said. "Maybe they're right."

"Victor dear, listen to me." I knelt down by his chair. "This is not right," I said calmly and clearly. "You are weak and tired all the time and I'm frightened every time you lose more blood. Someone has to look at you. Now I have a plan, so please just bear with me."

As Victor looked on, I took down a painting of an old barn from the wall, and started to wrap it in brown paper.

"Good grief. What are you up to now?" he asked.

"I'm going to see Dr. Earl Meyers in Toronto," I replied. "They call him the Rear Admiral. He was my brother-in-law's doctor. He's not only a prominent colon specialist, but he is also the president of the Ontario Medical Association." I tilted my head as I often did when I felt I was being clever.

"But you don't have an appointment," Victor said.

"I know. That's the chance I'll have to take. I'm going to walk in on his lunch hour. If I try to get an appointment his secretary will insist on a referral and we don't have one. Who's going to give us one when they think I'm being neurotic? Don't worry, Vitts. I'll go up to Toronto on the bus and I'll be back before you know it. Okay?"

"Whatever you say. I'm in your hands."

After lunch, Victor drove me to the bus station. He hugged me and handed me the painting as I boarded the bus and disappeared around the corner.

The waiting room was empty when I opened the door. There

was no sign of the secretary. My heart was pounding when I knocked on the door to Dr. Meyers's inner office and opened it. He was on the telephone. He showed little surprise, just motioned to me to sit down, said goodbye, and put down the telephone receiver.

I stood up. "Here, this is for you," I said, holding the painting out to him, "if you will look at my husband," I added. I was on the verge of crying.

"Hey, hey, what's this all about?" Dr. Meyers's tone was concerned and fatherly. I poured out the whole story.

"They're too quick to say it's radiation colitis," he said. "Bring him in. I want to have a look at him. My secretary will give you an appointment, Mrs. Newton. I'd like to see him as soon as possible." Sighing with relief, I thanked him and left his office. "I like the painting," he called after me. "I collect art. The fellow is good, very good. I'm looking forward to meeting him." He held the painting at arm's length.

I was elated when I told Victor the news but Victor had news of his own. While I was away, Dr. Ryder had called with an appointment for Victor to see a gastroenterologist. Dr. Norman Marcon would perform a colonoscopy, an investigation of the entire bowel to either exclude or confirm that the rectal bleeding was due to radiation colitis.

"Well, we had better do what Dr. Ryder suggests and take it from there. We can still see Dr. Meyers if we have to." I was delighted at the prospect of having two experts examine Victor. At least now we would find out for sure what was going on inside his colon. And about time too!

To get ready for the exam, Victor had to drink quantities of

Citromag, a purging liquid, and other fluids over a period of about a day and a half in order to clean out his bowel. Dr. Marcon performed the colonoscopy on Victor, who had been admitted as an out-patient at the Wellesley Hospital in Toronto. Afterwards, the nurse told him to get dressed and join me in the waiting room, until the doctor could speak to us. Victor felt a little weak, but otherwise glad that the ordeal was over. It had not been pleasant and had at times been painful.

"Having a scope with a lens attached to it up your ass is no fun," he told me later.

"Mr. Newton, I have good news and bad." Dr. Marcon held Victor's hand. I took the other one and waited. "We have found three polyps," the doctor said. "Two are benign and one is malignant. We often find these small, fleshy protrusions in the colons of people over the age of fifty. Most of them are harmless, however, some of them are malignant. This means, of course, that you will need an operation, a bowel resection. A surgeon will have to remove a portion of the bowel." Victor and I said nothing for a long moment.

Finally, Victor asked, "And the good news?"

"The good news is that we have found your cancer just in time. It has not grown out of the wall of the bowel and you will no doubt be cured. You are very lucky," the doctor said. "Very lucky. You can expect a full recovery. Now, do you have a surgeon in mind or would you like me to recommend one?"

"Dr. Earl Meyers. We have an appointment to see him on Thursday."

"Good. I'll give him a call then." Dr. Marcon shook hands with Victor. "He needs a good meal, Mrs. Newton."

"It's ready and waiting." I smiled. "Just have to heat it up."

"It's going to be okay, Vitts," I said. "You heard what Dr. Marcon said. 'We caught it in time'?"

"Thanks to you, sweetheart. If you hadn't persisted, if you had listened to the other doctors, the cancer could have spread and killed me." He nosed the car onto the highway in the direction of home.

"Want me to sing for you, Vitts?"

"Absolutely," he said as he patted my knee and sighed deeply.

On January 20, 1984, Victor was operated on for colon cancer.

"The operation was a success. I mean a total success," Dr. Meyers said. He was still wearing operating-room garb. He walked to the elevator with me. "We got it in time," he continued. He stopped and looked at me squarely. "He's cured."

"What about the colostomy?" I asked. "Did you have to make an artificial opening?"

"Oh, he didn't need one. It wasn't necessary, the cancer was high up in the bowel."

"Are you saying this cancer had nothing to do with the prostate? And it is not the cause of his pelvic pain?"

"Absolutely nothing. If he hadn't had prostate cancer, he would still have had colon cancer. You see, Mrs. Newton, prostate cancer invariably goes to the bone; and in terminal cases, to the lungs and the liver. I understand his prostate cancer is under control."

Dr. Meyers looked at his watch. "Gotta run. Your husband will be in recovery for a few hours. You can see him around four. Why don't you grab yourself some lunch?" He motioned towards the cafeteria and disappeared into the elevator.

"Your daughter is here to see you, Mr. Newton," the nurse smiled at him as Victor tried to raise his head.

"That's not my daughter." He held out his hand to me. "That's my beautiful young wife."

"Oh, I'm sorry, Mr. Newton." The nurse was blushing.

"That's okay," I reassured her. "We're used to it. I'm really not that much younger. It's Victor's grey hair that fools people."

"So Vitts. Dr. Meyers told me it was the earliest cancer he had ever removed. I'll bet you'll be skiing before the season is over." I brushed the hair from his forehead.

Two months to the day, Victor was skiing at Devil's Elbow a few miles west of Peterborough. He felt very good physically. He thanked God for the new life pouring into him. Skiing was one of Victor's passions, and he was grateful to be back on the hills again.

~

"Victor, look at this story in *The Toronto Star*. It's about a man seeking treatment for prostate cancer at a clinic in Texas. A doctor is giving him a drug made from human urine, which he gets from prisoners at a state institution."

"May I see that?" Victor looked at the photo of the man with the big grin. "Well, I'll be. . . . It's Kenny Burns."

"You know him?" I asked, looking over Victor's shoulder at the paper.

"I sure do. I haven't seen him in years. We did some bar-hopping during my freedom days."

"Your what?" I asked, teasing him.

"Well, you know I was a bachelor for five years before you caught me. No kidding, he's a great guy. You would like him."

"Why don't I find out?" I said. "I'm going up to Toronto to see Rob next week and I'll call Kenny Burns and invite him over. I would really like to hear more about his unconventional cancer treatment and his reasons for not taking radiation therapy."

The following week, while visiting Rob in Toronto, I called Kenny Burns. He was a big, extroverted, and likeable man. "God, I can't believe it," he said when we met at Rob's apartment. "Good old Vic. We'll get together when I finish these treatments. I'll be flying down to Texas this weekend."

"Why not a more conventional form of treatment?" I asked.

Kenny poured out his story. He hadn't been happy with the advice he got from doctors in Canada, he said. None of them could offer him any hope of recovery. They had proposed surgery as a way to slow the disease but Kenny had had enough of operations.

"That's when I heard about Dr. Maurice in Texas," he said, "and the wonderful results he was getting with his cancer treatments. My prostate cancer is in Stage D2, and has already spread to the bones. I felt I had nothing to lose by trying this treatment, except another twenty grand. That's what it's cost me so far with travel expenses included."

"Victor's cancer was diagnosed as Stage D1. It was found in one lymph node," I said. "He has done well on radiation."

"Give him these brochures on the serum, in case the cancer comes back; he may be interested. Look, I'm so glad you called. Give Vic my best. We'll get together soon." Kenny held my hand, with a mischievous look in his twinkling blue eyes. "Tell Vic I said he's a lucky old dog."

When he had gone, the room seemed empty, as if a big piece of furniture was missing. I watched from the window as Kenny made his way to his car. His raincoat swirled around him and his blond hair tossed in the late fall breeze. I couldn't hear him, but I sensed Kenny was whistling as he drove away into the night.

It was shortly after New Year's Day, 1986, when Kenny called from the Toronto General Hospital. "I'm paralyzed, Vic. The goddamn cancer has paralyzed me. I'll never walk again."

Victor and I drove to the hospital the following day. Kenny was depressed. Although we tried to console him, no matter what we said, the words seemed lame and useless. When Kenny spoke, it was apparent that he was consumed by the fear of death. He turned his sad eyes towards the window and kept them fixed on a vision that no one else could see. He died a week later, a day before his sixtieth birthday.

~

"You know, Vitts," I said. "I see life as a mountain with some people near the top and some near the bottom, but most of us about halfway," I said. "We meet people on the mountain, like Kenny, who fall off and are gone forever. But, however tenuous a hold we have, the rest of us cling to the mountain. We don't want to let go."

"Where do we go when we reach the top?" Victor asked.

"I guess we push off towards the light," I replied. "Maybe there's another mountain."

"Come here, sweetheart. You take on too much. You need a big hug." Victor held me for a long time. "Tell you what I'm going to do. You are staying in bed tomorrow and I'm fixing breakfast." Victor kept his promise and brought a tray of scrambled eggs, toast, marmalade, and a pot of tea. He surprised me by adding a bunch of red and white carnations purchased at the variety store when he bought the morning papers. The neighbour's cat, Max, followed him into the bedroom. Victor knew Max and I were best friends and that I would make a fuss over him.

"You've made me feel special, Vitts. It's a new year and I've been thinking this is going to be a free year, free from doctors and hospitals and illness. This year is for us. I'm going to do over that spare room and make it into a gallery for all those new paintings you are going to paint. What do you think?"

"I think it's a wonderful idea," he said as he took the tray from me. "All your ideas are wonderful."

"Oh, one more thing, Vitts."

"Yes?"

"I have a new motto. Want to hear it?"

"Absolutely, sweetheart."

"Remember the best and forget all the rest. What do you think?"

"Perfect. We'll put it into practice right away." He smiled as he carried the tray downstairs with Max, ever the opportunist on the lookout for crumbs of food and love, trailing behind him.

"I'll finish up here, Vitts." I brushed the last strokes of white paint on the wall and surveyed the new art room. "Looks great, huh? No curtains or drapes, just the white mini blinds. I can't wait to see the paintings on the wall. What do you think?"

"You've done a wonderful job. Hey, look at the time! I'm going to be late for the dentist. I'll probably be about an hour," Victor said. He raced down the stairs and out the door.

"Close your eyes before you come into the room," I yelled when I heard Victor return. "I hung some paintings and they look fabulous. Now you can open your eyes." I led him by the hand into the gallery. "Well?" I said waiting for an effusion of compliments.

"Very nice, angel. Very nice." Victor turned and walked into the bedroom and lay down on the bed. I followed him.

"Victor, what is it? Something is wrong. Are you ill?"

"The dentist says I have something on the back of my tongue and I should be seen by doctors at the Princess Margaret Hospital."

"My God, Victor. You never told me." I was shocked.

"I never knew it was there," he said. "I never felt anything. Now I suppose they'll cut my tongue out."

"Oh Victor, no! No, they won't. Now let's not panic. Come into the bathroom and let me look at it. The light is better there." He followed me in. I held his tongue with a Kleenex in one hand and a flashlight in the other.

"I see it, Vitts. It doesn't look threatening. You have a few deep crevices on your tongue. It could be an ulcer. From what I have read about oral cancers you don't have any of the usual obvious symptoms; but the dentist is right, we can't take chances. We have to check it out. I'll call the Princess Margaret Hospital and make an appointment for you. I know how worrying this is, and that's normal, but I have an instinct for these things and I think you are going to be okay. They can look at that sore spot on your ear, too. It's been bothering you for a long time."

"Good grief. I suppose they'll want to cut my ear off, too," Victor said.

"Hey, that's not a bad idea," I responded. "Then they can call you 'Vic Van Newton,' the mad artist of Peterborough!"

≈

"I don't think you have a malignancy here, Mr. Newton. However, I'd like to excise it to be absolutely sure. We can't be certain until we have it under a microscope." Dr. McGrail turned his attention to Victor's ear. "You do have a basal cell carcinoma on your left ear. It probably won't do much more than cause you a little irritation from time to time, but if you notice any change, such as a lump or thickening, then you must bring it to our attention. These little basal cell cancers are not as malignant as the melanomas, which are deadly if not caught early; nevertheless, you should avoid the sun or at least wear protective gear such as a hat, Mr. Newton. Especially on the golf course."

"Thank you, Doctor, I will," Victor said.

"You can come in on Monday and I'll do the surgery on Tuesday. My nurse will make the arrangements for you, Mr. Newton."

We returned to the hospital on Monday and headed for the admission office. Victor carried a travel bag and I carried a small slate board. We had been advised to bring one because Victor would have stitches in his tongue and would be unable to speak for a few days, thus the slate for communication. Suddenly Victor saw a familiar face near the elevator.

"Stan. It's been a long time," he said. He beamed and extended his hand to a tall, frail man with steel-blue eyes. Stan smiled broadly but did not speak. When he pointed to his throat, the reason for his silence became evident. Stan had lost his larynx to cancer. He quickly wrote a message on the notepad he was carrying, and before long had exchanged cancer stories with Victor. Stan was curious about the slate I was carrying. He wished us well and promised to keep in touch.

We were surprised to see Stan the following day. He had come to Victor's room just as the surgeon was giving us the report on Victor's biopsy. Stan waited for us to have a free moment.

"No malignancy. You can go home today whenever you feel up to it." Dr. McGrail sat on the edge of the bed, the pathologist's report in his hands.

"What was it, Doctor?" Victor asked, becoming aware of the stitches on the back of his tongue.

"An inflamed lesion, not unlike a mouth ulcer; somewhat calcified, but otherwise benign. The stitches will dissolve in three or four days. You can call for an appointment in a few weeks. I'll see you then." The doctor shook Victor's hand, nodded to me, and left.

As soon as he had gone, Victor got out of bed, kissed and

hugged me, and began to dress. We had forgotten Stan until he extended his hand and showed Victor his note of congratulations, wished us well, and said goodbye. We watched him walk away, shoulders slumped.

"I think it was bad timing. I mean, it must be difficult for him to see and be part of good news when his own cancer has recurred," I said.

We were on our way out of the hospital when we saw Stan again. He was sitting near the exit, almost as if he were waiting for us. Victor talked to him for a few minutes and Stan wrote his replies on his little notepad.

"Here, Stan, you take this." Victor handed him the slate board, wished him well, and promised to call.

Out in the parking lot Victor slammed his fist down hard on the top of the car.

"Damn it! Why did I do that?"

"What? What is it, Victor?" I ran around the car. "Are you all right?"

"I gave Stan the goddamn slate. Did you see his face, the look in his eyes like a wounded animal? What the hell was I thinking of? I should never have done that."

"Victor, calm down. Listen to me. It's not your fault Stan lost his larynx. If he's feeling down and depressed, what are you supposed to do? Say you're sorry because you didn't lose your tongue? It's human nature for people to feel better when someone shares their pain and trouble, yes, and cancer, too. Whoever coined the phrase 'misery loves company' knew what they were talking about because it's true. But don't you ever feel bad about feeling good, Vitts! Stan was down before you met him yesterday, and he will have to work it out himself. You gave him the slate because it was better than the notepad and because you didn't need it. Don't reproach yourself, sweetheart. You would never hurt anybody. I know it and God knows it and so does Stan."

Victor had tears on his cheeks. "I sure love you," he said. "Come on. It's been a long day. I want to go home with my wife."

The End of the Journey

The distinction between stages of disease is an arbitrary one. There is no single moment when Victor's cancer ceased to be something he lived with and became, instead, something that was killing him. It was killing him from the beginning and he lived with it until the end. Still, there is some reason to divide the experience into periods. There was a time when Victor lived a more or less normal life despite the disease, and it was followed by a period that was not like normal life at all, when we understood that his life itself was nearing its end. There was no defining moment that separated one period from the other, but they were nonetheless different.

When prostate cancer spreads, or metastasizes, to the spine and other vital organs, the patient is almost invariably under the supervision of his doctor, who may recommend palliative care. At this point, the patient's needs will be complex, meaning that he has a variety of physical and emotional needs that require the attention of professional people. Hospice is a volunteer organization whose members provide palliative care at home – they treat the patient with the best care possible but without hope of curing him. Trained health care professionals and volunteer visitors apply their unique expertise in a hospital setting as well, if that is what the patient asks for. The aim of the hospice team, either at home or in hospital, is to provide care and comfort to the terminally ill patient and support to his loved ones. The emotional state of the patient is their primary concern, next to keeping him as pain-free as possible. Families should enquire about the hospice services in their own community as they may differ from the services offered in other communities.

"Everything went well, Mr. Newton. You can go home tomorrow."

Dr. Buckspan, one of the senior urologists at Mount Sinai Hospital in Toronto, had performed the procedure on Victor a half dozen times in the past three years. Known as a urethral dilation and cystoscopy, it involved inserting an instrument into the urethra through the penis, which stretched (or dilated) the urethra and allowed a visual examination of the bladder. The procedure was necessary in Victor's case because the radiation treatments to the prostate caused scar tissue to form in the urethra. The scar tissue caused a stricture or tightening of the urethra, which slowed the flow of urine, making it difficult or impossible for Victor to empty his bladder completely. Victor would have an urgent need to pee but then have difficulty expelling the urine: it might take him as many as three minutes to empty his bladder. After the cystoscopy and stretching, which was performed painlessly under light sedation, Victor would be able to urinate normally for about six to eight months. Then the urethra would tighten up again. Victor never complained about having to undergo this procedure. He was always grateful to Dr. Buckspan for his help in relieving him of the agony of getting up at night with an aching bladder and then having to strain to achieve even a halting, dribbling flow.

"There is no other way to describe it, except as sheer torment," Victor told me.

I returned to the Mount Sinai Hospital after a short jaunt to the Eaton Centre a few blocks away. "What do you think, Vitts?"

"You're wearing a hat. I haven't seen you in a hat before."

"I know. That's why I bought it. It was on sale, but mostly I bought it because it's just like the one Ingrid Bergman wore when she gave that tearful goodbye to Bogey in *Casablanca*. So, what do you think?"

"Strange but beautiful. Will you wear it to bed some time?"

I laughed and playfully placed the hat on Victor's head. "Oh, what's this?" I nudged Victor as four white-coated young men advanced upon our corner of the room.

"Mr. Newton, my name is Dr. Smith and these are my associates. How are you feeling?"

"Fine. I'm going home tomorrow," Victor said. He was feeling uneasy about the sudden appearance of these doctors around his bed.

"We don't want to alarm you, Mr. Newton; however, your

lung X-rays have revealed a lesion on the lower lobe of your left lung. We would like you to stay in the hospital until Dr. Goldberg, a very good lung man, can see you tomorrow. He will want to do a bronchoscopy and remove a small piece of tissue for biopsy. With your history of prostate cancer, we don't want to take any chances. We have to determine if this is a primary or metastatic disease. It could be neither, but we want to be sure. Have a good night, Mr. Newton."

The young interns looked from Victor's anxious face to mine, turned on their soft-soled shoes, and seemingly floated out of the room, their white coats billowing behind them.

Victor closed his eyes and took a deep breath. "I know, sweetheart, we're walking through the fire, again," he said as he squeezed my hand.

The bronchoscopy was very uncomfortable. A scope was placed down Victor's throat and into the bronchial tube. A piece of tissue was snipped for the biopsy. Victor never complained. The possibility of lung cancer posed a far greater threat than any test.

Dr. Goldberg gave him the results: an adenocarcinoma. He would operate the following day and remove the lower lobe of Victor's left lung. This drastic news was numbing. It all happened so fast that we could hardly grasp it. Victor accepted the news rather passively. "What can we do, sweetheart? If they say I have cancer in my lung and I need an operation, I can't argue with them. They are the experts."

I was not so sure. I went to see Dr. Goldberg in his office on the second floor for a further explanation. Then I talked to the urologist, Dr. Buckspan, who was concurring with Dr. Goldberg.

"I'm not satisfied that this is a primary cancer," I said. "I would like more tests, more proof."

"We can do an MRI, magnetic resonance imaging, to determine if there is any cancer from the prostate in the bones. We will send him over to the Toronto General Hospital, where they have the machine. It's a very sophisticated machine, and picks up what the bone scan misses."

I was satisfied and returned to Victor.

~

While I was out of the room, the veterinarian at the pet hospital where we boarded Cleo had called to say that Cleo was failing fast. He said it was simply her age. She was twelve years old and dogs of her breed rarely lived longer than that.

"You go to her," Victor pleaded. "There is nothing you can do here. If I have surgery, I'll be in recovery most of the day. You may be able to help Cleo." We kissed goodbye and wiped away each other's tears.

I was at the veterinary hospital a few hours later with a taxi, a station wagon. The vet said Cleo's condition was very serious; she was near death. With my permission he would put her to sleep.

"No, I'll take her home. If she's going to die, she will die at home," I said. Two men carried Cleo out and put her in the back of the taxi. I got in beside her and soothed her, talking to and petting her. When we arrived at the house the driver said he could not help because he had a bad back, so I dragged the heavy dog off the tailgate onto the snow-covered ground, falling with her.

It was mid-January and the blizzard that had been building all day was now much worse. The street was empty. After paying the driver, I dragged Cleo to the back of the house. "Come on, Cleo, old girl. You can do it." I coaxed the sick animal to her doghouse, and with all the strength she could muster she pulled herself up and into the house. I got some dry straw from the basement and pushed it in all around her to keep her warm. Next I boiled a mixture of minced beef and rice and fed her small amounts every twenty minutes. Cleo improved by the hour. She was very weak but she was recovering her strength.

It was around 11:00 p.m. when I made one last check on her before I went to bed. Down on my knees in the snow with a flashlight, I was suddenly aware of someone in the house and turned to see Victor standing in the doorway.

"Oh my God, Victor!"

"I'm sorry, sweetheart, I didn't mean to startle you, but I called to you and you couldn't hear me out here. I telephoned and I guess you were with Cleo. How is she?"

"Cleo's going to be fine. Let's get inside. I want to know about you." I was lightheaded. I had not eaten all day so I put the kettle on for tea and listened to Victor's incredible story.

"After you left, they sent me for the MRI test and found cancer in my left clavicle. Apparently it's metastatic disease from the original prostate cancer, and they've now concluded that the lesion in my lung is metastatic cancer also. Dr. Buckspan and Dr. Goldberg had a little conference and cancelled the surgery. They sent me home with a prescription for a new hormone drug to combat the cancer. Dr. Buckspan says

I have to take it without fail, as it will stop the cancer in the lung from spreading."

"In other words, this is not a primary cancer as they first suspected."

I had *The Merck Manual* open to the section dealing with lung cancer and I had the cancer book, *Choices,* open to prostate cancer and metastatic disease. "You see, Vitts," I explained, "when you have a cancer metastasized from another site as you do, then it is not lung cancer, it is prostate cancer gone to the lung, and it progresses differently. It's the same when a woman's breast cancer metastasizes to the lung, or another person's bowel cancer metastasizes to the lung. The primary site in your case is still the prostate, just as the primary site in those other cases is the breast or bowel."

"What about the liver?" Victor asked. "The man in the next bed to me had liver cancer."

"Primary liver cancer is extremely rare," I said, looking up liver cancer in my reference books. "Cancer in the liver usually means the cancer has spread or metastasized from another site. Almost any cancer can spread to the liver."

Victor closed the books. "My poor angel, you're trembling. What you've been through this day! Come on, let's go to bed. We're both exhausted."

"You go on up," I said. "I want to check on Cleo one more time."

The big dog was warm and content to be where she was. I looked up at the clear night sky. All was calm, the storm had abated. "Thank you, God, for bringing them home," I said. I took a deep breath and choked back the tears.

~

The following day when we were both rested we tried to put everything in perspective.

"No surgery, just carry on with a bottle of pills," Victor said. "Seems rather strange and quiet after all the drama of the last few days. I feel as though I caught the brass ring, but I can't pull it free."

"Well, that's not acceptable, Vitts. I'm calling the Princess Margaret Hospital. I'm sure they will want to see you. After all, you are one of their star patients. An eight-year survivor of two major cancers." I dialled the number of the hospital and asked for Dr. Hawkins, an oncologist in the urology department.

Victor felt better already. He knew from experience that between me and the Princess Margaret Hospital, all that was humanly and medically possible was being done for him.

A week later, we found ourselves in familiar surroundings back in Clinic J at the Princess Margaret Hospital.

"We sent for your tests done at Mount Sinai, Mr. Newton, and have confirmed their finding of metastatic prostate cancer in your left lung. You also have multiple bone metastases, which is a common occurrence in progressive prostate cancer," Dr. Hawkins said. He looked at the X-rays. With a small wand he pointed to a spot on the left clavicle (collar-bone) and another on the lower spine. "We can treat the bone metastasis with radiation and the lung lesion with hormone drug therapy. I believe Dr. Buckspan prescribed the medication for you. How are you tolerating it, Mr. Newton? I see by your chart that you did not tolerate the previous hormone drug therapy very well."

Victor had a sinking feeling. "Is this the same kind of drug? If it is, I won't take it. I would rather die than go through that again."

"It is a hormone drug, but a different drug. Why don't you try it? I'll start you on small doses and gradually increase the dosage as your body adapts. It has been shown to stop the spread of prostate cancer very successfully, Mr. Newton. If you can return on Friday to Planning on the first floor, they will give you your radiation treatments and I will see you in four weeks."

The following Friday, Victor's shoulder and spine were marked to guide the radiation beam. "Turn this way, Mr. Newton." The technician moved him into position and Victor yelped loudly – he felt a piercing pain in his left collar-bone.

"I think I must have pulled that shoulder playing golf," he said, wincing. The radiologist proceeded with the treatment. It lasted only a minute.

"You should have your doctor in Peterborough look at that shoulder, Mr. Newton."

"Oh, I think it will be all right. Nothing a little more golf won't cure," he joked.

But the pain worsened so that by the time we reached home Victor could only climb into bed. I called the doctor.

X-rays at the local hospital revealed a tiny fracture to his left collar-bone. Victor was convinced his golf swing was the cause, but when Dr. Hawkins was informed, he suggested that Victor return to the Princess Margaret Hospital for further X-rays and radiation treatment. Dr. Hawkins explained that prostate cancer metastasizes to the bone, weakening the bone, sometimes causing tiny fractures.

~

It was late spring and the terrible uncertainty and fear that filled the winter months began to fade. Victor felt well and was anxious to play golf again. "If we could just sell a few paintings, we could get you a golf membership, Vitts, but when we sell a painting at three hundred dollars that cost two hundred dollars to make, there really isn't much left over."

I had called every corporation in the city and had sent out brochures describing Victor's work to every doctor and lawyer, hoping to make a few sales, all to no avail. It hurt whenever we had to sell our possessions to make ends meet. When there was nothing left to sell, we bartered paintings.

"Where are friends when you need them?" Victor asked rhetorically.

"You have some wonderful, loyal friends here in Peterborough, Vitts, and I think they love you."

"Oh yeah, but who loves who around here?" he teased.

"Well, I love you, and Cleo loves you and you love me and Cleo . . ." Victor's bitterness never lasted very long. He was quick to recover, resilient and forgiving. Whenever we argued, I would bring him a peace offering of a cup of hot chocolate and a kiss and all would be forgiven and forgotten.

"Your kisses make me forget my name," he told me. "Kissing you, sweetheart, is like drinking a glass of hot rum."

"Vitts, you are such a romantic," I said kissing him again. "In that case I'm going to make you drunk with my kisses." Whenever we fooled around, Cleo would bark and wag her tail.

～

"What luck! I can hardly control my joy, Vitts. Four paintings in one week! That's the most we have ever sold in such a short time. Thank God for Canadian General Electric!"

Victor put the last stroke of varnish on a painting and laid it flat to dry.

"They love your work because they recognize all the lakes and woods around here. You're pretty well known at the plant. They refer to you as the 'Kawartha Artist.' That last couple who were here yesterday told me that whenever someone comes up for a forty-year service award the others tell him to go to the Newton Gallery on Chamberlain Street because Mr. Newton is the best."

"You sweetheart you. Stop flattering me and tell me what you have planned for the money. We could use a new lawnmower."

"No lawnmowers," I said emphatically. "The old one is good enough for another year. We're getting you a golf membership for next season and there is absolutely no use in arguing about it because I sent the cheque this morning."

I went into the kitchen to make tea while Victor sat in the living room and waited for me. He thought about the first time we sat in the same living room. It was in December. He had been so very ill that he hadn't expected to live through the winter. The room had been cold but we were reluctant to put the heat above sixty degrees Fahrenheit because of the cost, so we had wrapped ourselves in coats and blankets all through that first winter.

Now the rooms were filled with pine furniture, decorator

rugs, and antique lamps. Flowers and paintings were every-where. And the room was warm.

I had always wanted a queen-size bed and Victor surprised me with one on my birthday. He never told me how he paid for it. In no time I had it covered with a light and airy duvet and a half dozen colourful cushions. I covered the windows in white lace curtains and hung a huge abstract painting I had asked him to do especially for the bedroom in swirling graduating colours of the faintest to the darkest shades of purple. The wavy swirls made my head sway and I called the painting *Dreamscape*.

I called Cleo into the house for her afternoon visit.

"I'm worried about her, Vitts. She had an awful time getting up."

"She's old, sweetheart. In people years she's probably about eighty."

"Oh, I never believed that theory," I said, as I laced my tea with sugar. "Cleo is twelve and that's all there is to it. But twelve is old for a dog, I agree." Cleo lay down with her head between her big paws and looked from me to Victor depend-ing on who was speaking. Finally she sighed deeply and fell asleep.

The following week she had a stroke. She could not get up. "It's time, sweetheart," Victor said, as I petted the big dog's head and talked soothingly to her.

With tears streaming down my face I told him, "I want the vet to come here. I don't want Cleo taken away and frightened. I promised her I would never give her away again and I won't."

"Okay, sweetheart. I'll call him," Victor said, as he cleared his throat.

Dr. Muise came into the yard and spoke to Cleo. Cleo knew him and was not afraid. He left Victor and me alone with her to say our goodbyes. Victor patted her on the head and choked up as he said, "So long, old girl. Thanks for the love and loyalty all these years." Then he went inside and left me alone with her.

"I love you, Cleo," I said. "I'll think of you as you were in your youth, filled with the love of life. Love never dies, Cleo," I said, hugging her around the neck. Cleo never took her big brown eyes off me until I was inside the house.

Dr. Muise knocked on the door. "It's over," he said. "She's in the pickup truck. I'll take her away now. She never felt a thing. In fact, she licked my hand as I put the needle in." The doctor had tears on his cheeks. "Well, Mrs. Newton, you gave her another spring and summer. She was all but gone last January." He walked to the truck and drove away.

I know it was my imagination, but I thought I heard a soft *woof, woof* before I closed the door.

❧

"I'll get it." I bounded for the ringing telephone. "Oh, my goodness! Hal Bergman! It's been years. How are you?"

Hal had emigrated from Germany in the 1960s, bringing his young wife and son to begin a new life in Canada. He was the real estate agent who sold our house when I was married to my first husband, Allan. My brother Joe worked with him learning the business. Joe and Hal were best friends. Hal had done very well in real estate and was now the devoted father of four grown-up children.

"My daughter is going to Trent University and I was visiting her so I looked up your number," he said. "I was talking to Joseph and he told me about your husband's cancer. How is he?"

"Fine. He's right here. He still has to take drug treatment but he plays golf and paints. We're very grateful for his present health. You should bring Helga down some Sunday to see his paintings."

"I'd like that," Hal said. "But I will probably be doctoring myself. I may have cancer too."

"What makes you say that? What symptoms do you have?"

"Bleeding. At first I thought I had haemorrhoids, but now I am experiencing pain around my liver."

"How long have you had these symptoms?" I took on the role of the doctor whenever someone questioned me about medical matters. I couldn't help it. It was natural for me and although I never went beyond my limits, I did encourage a lot of people to seek professional help.

"I guess it must be about six months." Hal's voice quavered a little.

"I would urge you to see a doctor right away, Hal. Don't put it off any longer. The fact that you are talking to me about it tells me that you are seriously concerned. Now promise we'll keep in touch. Victor and I are here for you. Call whenever you feel the need." He said goodbye with a promise to stay in touch.

Three weeks later Joe called to say that Hal had been operated on for colon cancer, which had spread to his liver. He had been given less than six months to live. The doctors said chemotherapy would not be prescribed because it would be useless – the cancer had progressed too far.

~

Victor continued to play golf. He began to experience back pain and treated it successfully with Tylenol. Although he was not due for reassessment at the Princess Margaret Hospital until November, he returned there to have a small basal cell carcinoma removed from the back of his hand in July. All went well and it healed.

My son, Rob, had informed me that his father had been diagnosed with bladder cancer and was taking treatment at the Princess Margaret Hospital. On one of our visits to the hospital I saw Allan coming out of the radiation treatment room. It was the first time I had seen him since our divorce more than seventeen years before.

"Fancy meeting you here," Allan said when he saw me.

"Hello, Allan. This is Victor." The two men shook hands and eyed one another. They each soon concluded that there was nothing threatening about the other and exchanged cancer stories.

Allan suddenly and surprisingly began to cry. Tears rolled down his cheeks. He'd had some heavy chemotherapy and was wearing a winter tuque to cover the baldness caused by the drugs. Victor and I put our arms around his frail frame, reassuring and comforting him. We walked him to the car. By the time we got there Allan had composed himself and lit a cigarette. He had always been a heavy smoker and would not give up the habit. Rob said his father's doctor told him that smoking had been a factor contributing to the development of the bladder cancer.

I gave Allan our telephone number before we said goodbye and his tears fell again. "Nobody calls me any more," he said. He seemed like a little boy, sad and lost.

"Don't worry, Allan, I'll call you and you can call Victor and me any time, night or day, whenever you want to talk." I kissed him and we drove away feeling down and sad.

~

On the way home to Peterborough we stopped in to see Hal and Helga who lived in Scarborough. Hal had been to Greece to receive a controversial treatment from a doctor there who claimed to have halted the progress of some cancers and even to have cured them with his injections. The doctor would not reveal what was in the magic serum.

Hal told Victor and me that he had seen people from other countries, mostly from the United States, being helped by the treatment and he had seen a great improvement in his own cancer. He asked me to place my hand over his liver and feel the tumours, how they were shrinking. We were shocked to hear Hal talk this way when, in fact, he had deteriorated badly. He had become so nearly skeletal that we hardly recognized him. I told Victor later that Hal's liver felt like a bunch of grapes.

"Here is another cure I'm taking," Hal said. He produced a large plastic bottle crudely labelled and filled with a thick black liquid. "Take one tablespoonful and leave under the tongue for five minutes, three times a day," were the instructions.

Hal said he was willing to try anything now. His doctors had refused him conventional treatment, saying it would be of no use to him. "They told me to go home and put my things in order," he said. He suddenly jumped up at the sound of a shrill bell.

"It's time for my cancer-cure medicine," he said. He made his way to the bathroom. Victor and Helga and I sat there not speaking for several minutes.

"I bought ten pounds of carrots today," Helga said thoughtfully. "I'm making juice. They say it's good for cancer, too."

~

A few weeks later Rob came to Peterborough by bus. His car was in the garage and he wanted Victor and me to drive him to Lindsay where his father had been hospitalized for the past few weeks. Rob's Aunt Dorothy, who was looking after her brother Allan, had called to say his dad was gravely ill.

"We'll stay here in the lounge," I said when we arrived at the hospital. "I'm no longer a part of that family, Rob, and Allan's sisters will be with him. We'll be right here if you need us." I watched Rob disappear into the elevator, only to return in minutes, tears streaming down his cheeks.

"Mom, Dad looks pretty bad. Can you and Vic come up with me?" We followed Rob down the long corridor to Allan's room.

Dorothy was holding her brother's hand. The bed was raised to a forty-five-degree angle. Allan was in a blue hospital gown with a sheet folded in two and placed over his middle leaving his legs and feet exposed. His arms lay limply at his sides. His head was tilted back, his eyes wide open and rolling, and his mouth agape as he struggled for each and every breath.

"He's dying, Mom. Come in with me." Rob took my hand and led me to the bed. Standing there, watching the life slowly ebb from my son's father, I didn't know what to say. Allan was a quiet man who told corny jokes when he said anything at all.

"I'm here, Allan," I finally said. "It's me, Audie, and Rob. We're right here." Victor and Allan's sister and her husband looked on the deathbed scene with curious silence. Rob wept quietly and Allan gasped loudly.

I remembered something a nurse had told me, that the hearing of a dying individual was the last of the senses to fail. So I said, "Allan, do you remember that little joke you used to tell me so often, about the man who bought a new fedora and his wife asked him if it was for Dora and he said, No, it's for me? Well, I finally got that joke," I said, squeezing his hand.

Rob looked at me and Dorothy raised her eyebrows. Victor smiled. He knew I had a good reason for whatever it was I felt I had to say to Allan and that's all that mattered. The nurse whispered that Allan could linger for some hours and she suggested we get something to eat. As we all filed out I hung back for a minute. Allan took one last breath and died.

Rob stayed in Lindsay to help with the funeral arrangements. Later, Joe called to say that Hal had died hours before Allan on the same day, July 20, 1990.

≈

Victor's pain eased a little but he was reluctant to pick up anything heavy, even a bag of groceries, because he was constantly aware of the fragility of his spine. The challenge we faced was to keep the level of pain tolerable as the cancer ate at his bones and the tumours threatened to break them open. Because golf was out of the question now, we decided to plant an English garden.

Victor was enthusiastic about the project. He completely lost his depression and was his cheerful self again.

"It's spring, sweetheart," Victor said. "I saw Mrs. Robin building her nest in the blue spruce this morning." He stood at the window watching the yard come to life.

My newest pet squirrel, Baby, was chasing the neighbour's cat, Max, around the holly bush, and a variety of birds had returned to take up residence in old nests, busying themselves with spring cleaning. Everything turned green and buds sprouted overnight.

The yard was deep and private with a high steel fence at the end against the brick wall of another building. In summer the fence was covered with leafy vines. We had built a sun-deck on the back of the house the previous year. I had placed white summer furniture on the deck along with a variety of terra cotta pots and planters filled with geraniums, marigolds, and hibiscus plants. The deck was a mass of colour. Now Victor looked at the fruit trees he had planted five years before, which zigzagged through the middle of the yard along with a number of flowering bushes, and imagined the whole yard as a show-place of summer flowers.

He set his artist's eye to the task of arranging flower-beds.

"Looks wonderful," I said when I looked at the plans he had sketched. "I can hardly wait."

Victor took the spade and dug out the edges of the beds,

giving them size and shape, and I turned over the sod, shaking out the good earth and discarding the grass. The beds were to be five by ten feet on one side and five by twenty feet in a kidney shape on the other side.

Victor planted forty varieties of flowers, some of which he started from seed inside the house. With compost and peat moss we nourished the earth and gently watered the seeds.

While we waited for the flowers to bloom Victor was back at the Princess Margaret Hospital. This time he received more radiation to his right rib cage and, as a trial, one chemotherapy treatment. It was the first time he had received chemotherapy and it was discontinued immediately because it had no effect on the progress of his disease. He lost a little hair, but not much.

Victor didn't talk about his cancer any more. He was totally immersed in his garden, waiting and watching for new blooms to appear. The packets the seeds came in – with pictures of the flowers on them – had mysteriously disappeared, and I wondered if he had thrown them out intentionally so that we could enjoy the excitement of discovering new flowers and guess what each one was as it sprang from the ground.

"Look, Vitts," I would say as I dashed from one flower to the other. "What do you suppose this one is?" Then Victor would get out all the flower books and try to identify it.

"A Mexican sunflower. Wow! Look at it. It must be six feet high at least." He would take his coffee and walk in the garden every morning searching for and identifying new blossoms.

~

It was the end of August and the garden was in full bloom.
Except for the carnations, everything else had arrived. Delicate
roses in both pale and strong shades of red and yellow. Asters,
nicotiana, Shasta daisies, snapdragons, lobelia, and dwarf
mixed stocks. Columbines, marigolds, cornflowers, sweetpeas,
and, of course, Victor's beloved cosmos. He loved all the
flowers but he loved the cosmos best. They grew tall, light, and
airy and when they swayed in the breeze they swayed together.
Their brilliant heads of red, pink, and white were often topped
by a monarch butterfly. The garden was a success. Neighbours
often dropped by to enjoy it. They had helped identify some
of the flowers.

"How do you feel today, Vitts?" I asked, sitting on the deck
in the sunshine.

"I feel hungry and sexy," he said, pulling me onto his knee.

"You know, Vitts, you amaze me. If I didn't know you, I would
never guess you had cancer. I just want you to know that I think
you are remarkable. You're my hero," I said.

"Don't cry, sweetheart. I'm not going anywhere. I'm staying
right here with you. You just keep giving me that loving medicine of yours." We walked the length of the garden again with
old Max trailing behind us.

"You made a little paradise for us, Vitts," I said, holding onto
his arm, feeling the warmth and love he so easily and generously gave.

~

It was September 1991. Victor was back at the Princess
Margaret Hospital for more radiation to his spine, which had

become unbearably painful. He also received distressing news. Many more new sites showed metastasis; seven vertebrae and many ribs on both sides, the left shoulder-blade and breastbone, his pelvis and some facial bones. There was nothing more they could do. His spine had received all the radiation they could safely give him. They radiated it one last time to lessen the pain and sent him home with a prescription for Dilaudid (morphine) and a follow-up appointment in another six weeks. It was near Thanksgiving. Victor knew it was a matter of months before his body would succumb completely to the ravages of the cancer. I kept the girls and the rest of the family informed. At this time, Victor was still remarkably mobile as long as his pain was under control. He had a fair appetite and was still sexually potent. He even continued to paint for a few hours each day.

Thanksgiving was, however, particularly sad because he knew it would be his last. He grew despondent. A few old friends came by and tried to comfort him, to no avail. He rarely smiled again.

A few days after Thanksgiving, Victor made two appointments; one with Mr. Vandermey at Little Lake Cemetery and the other with his lawyer, Mr. Coros.

Walking the one flight of stairs to Mr. Coros's office was difficult and painful. Victor had to rest partway. In Mr. Coros's office he made some drastic changes to his will.

"It's all up to you now," he said, as we drove to the cemetery where he would choose his final resting place.

Victor and I had always admired the beautiful old cemetery on the edge of Little Lake in the heart of Peterborough. We often drove through on its winding roads admiring the old stones and older trees. Victor had painted a picture of the charming little cemetery chapel. Once, when we were driving slowly by an old tombstone inscribed "John J. Crowe," a big crow had landed on it. We looked at one another. Victor usually kept his camera in the car, at the ready, but this time the camera was not there. He had forgotten it.

Mr. Vandermey showed us two gravesites. One was in an open area and the other was beneath a big maple tree not far from the lake.

"I like this one, Vitts." I leaned against the old tree.

"Let's look at the other one," Victor said, making his way to the open area.

"It's going to be a double depth; I'm going to be here too," I reminded him. It was fall and the leaves were being tossed this way and that.

When he reached the second gravesite he turned and looked back at me where I was standing beneath the maple tree. He paused for a long minute. Where he would be buried mattered to him and he took his time, just as he would if he were making any major purchase. Finally he said, "Yes, that's the one, sweetheart, where you are standing, beneath the maple tree."

A sudden gust of wind whipped at his coat and smoothed his hair away from his forehead as he made his way back to the sanctuary of the tree and my arms.

Later, over dinner, he told me he felt good about the day, that he had taken care of two important items that could no longer be put off. Victor slept peacefully that night while I lay awake, remembering him as he stood in the cemetery looking back at me with the wind in his pale face, his quiet courage shining through. Muffling my sobs I turned away from him. Consumed by my own unbearable pain, I prayed for sleep.

~

One day Victor brought home from the library a book entitled *Recalled by Life*. It was written by Anthony J. Sattilaro, M.D., a Philadelphia doctor, and it was the personal story of his recovery from prostate cancer. "I'll read this right after dinner," I said.

"I knew you would. I can't wait to hear your opinion." Victor smiled to himself knowing I would want to try anything that sounded reasonable and credible.

Because of the increasing pain in his back Victor could no longer sit for long periods and soon lost interest in television. He usually retired to the upstairs bedroom after dinner where he read his library books and I brought him tea and reported on the program I was watching or a news item I thought might interest him. I wanted to buy a small colour television for him. Victor insisted there were more important ways to spend any extra dollars we might have. The kitchen roof was leaking, which bothered him immensely. It was never repaired, only patched.

On this evening I went upstairs, lay on the bed beside him, and read Dr. Sattilaro's story.

In 1978 the doctor had been diagnosed with prostate cancer metastasized to the bone, spine, shoulder, skull, and breastbone. He was forty-seven years old. Feeling he had nothing to lose, he listened to the advice of a couple of young hitchhikers he had picked up. They encouraged him to try a macrobiotic diet of brown rice and steamed vegetables, beans, and seaweed. He tried it. Although he found the diet bland and unpalatable, he began to feel better.

In 1981 he underwent a sixth and final bone scan. No sign of cancer was found anywhere in his body. He was diagnosed by his physician to be in complete remission.

"So what do you think?" Victor asked.

"I think we'll give it a try. It worked for him. It should work for you," I replied.

"I knew you would want to try it." Victor smiled. "It can't hurt. Besides, I love rice, especially brown rice," he said. I boiled enough brown rice for several days, placing large bowls in the refrigerator. It was supposed to be effective hot or cold. I served it to Victor both ways, always accompanied by steamed vegetables.

After two weeks he was getting tired of the bland food and his bone pain was much worse. One morning, while he was in the shower, I called the Methodist Hospital in Philadelphia and asked to speak to Dr. Sattilaro. I was told they did not have a Dr. Sattilaro on staff. The operator switched me to Administration. A gentle voice told me that Dr. Sattilaro had died of prostate cancer in 1989.

Victor looked at his breakfast. "What, no brown rice?"

"Well, Vitts, I was thinking. You really should have protein while your body is fighting disease. Common sense tells me you can't possibly get all your nutrients from brown rice, or any other colour of rice for that matter."

"Whew," Victor sighed loudly. "Thank God! What a relief!" He smiled. "Pass the chili sauce, please. In that case, I wouldn't mind one of your fabulous pot roasts for dinner, the way you make it with the red wine." He smothered his scrambled eggs with chili sauce and grinned.

I never told him about the call to Philadelphia, but I felt somehow he knew. Nothing more was said about Dr. Sattilaro or brown rice.

~

The pain worsened and Victor couldn't sleep. When he lay on his back he said he felt as though there were a couple of golf balls under him, and because the cancer was growing in his left rib cage, he was unable to lie on that side. He rarely sat downstairs any more except for his meals. I would follow him to the bedroom and massage his back with a cooling lotion.

"Place your hands on my stomach, sweetheart. You really do have healing hands." Victor was serious about this and I would use my hands in a slow gathering motion over his abdomen.

"Now I am collecting all the pain," I said softly, and with a quick brush of my hand I would announce that I had swept the pain away.

"That feels better," Victor would say with conviction.

A few days later, I applied a new product, Hot Ice, to Victor's tortured spine. "Can you describe the pain?" I asked.

"Well, if you were to open me up and pour boiling water inside and close me again, that's what it feels like."

I raised my hand to my mouth. "Oh, my poor darling, how awful. There has to be something we can do." The pain medication gave some relief and the Hot Ice helped to cool his skin, but until he received more radiation, there was little else I could think of.

"We could try figs." Victor looked serious. "I was reading about a man in the Old Testament who had a bad back and they placed boiled figs on it and made him better." Victor watched me to gauge my reaction.

"I'll get some tomorrow, Vitts." I put my arms around him and buried my face in his shoulder.

"Don't worry, sweetheart," he said. "If the figs don't work, we can always eat them. I like figs."

"Oh, Vitts, you always make me laugh," I said, drying my tears.

The fig poultices did little more than offer temporary relief. I increased the dosage of pain medication. This, unfortunately, caused constipation. However, for all his pain and discomfort, Victor was still on his feet. Whenever he was feeling defeated, I would remind him that the cancer was not in his vital organs, and that some prostate cancers that have metastasized to the bone don't go to the vital organs for years.

"You make me feel better, sweetheart. Just keep talking to me like that. Don't let me give up."

"You won't, Vitts, you're not a quitter," I said.

It was the end of October and there was a noticeable chill in the air. "Hey! If we're going to plant tulips we had better get started." Victor sat in the lawn chair at the end of the garden. I put his woolen tuque on his head and wrapped a blanket around him. He held the bag of tulip bulbs on his lap.

"Now, Vitts, when I make the hole, you drop one in."

"Over there, sweetheart. We should have a dozen red and a dozen yellow here." Victor's artistic eye was painting the garden in an array of colour again.

"I think we will mix the rest," he said, as he dropped the bulbs into the holes and I covered them over with the rich dark earth. "It will be a beautiful spring showing," he said triumphantly.

I looked up at him from my kneeling position in the garden and for the first time I noticed how frail he had become. It suddenly struck me like a blow to the stomach that he would not see the tulips bloom. I resisted the urge to wail and scream, to let go all the hurt and emotion walled up for so long. Instead I swallowed hard, stood up, and put my arms around him. "I love you so much, my hero," I said. A brisk wind circled the garden and whipped the fallen leaves in a chilling reminder that winter was on the way.

The following morning Victor could not raise his head. The pain was agonizing. "Victor, what is it?" I leapt out of bed and hurried around to his side.

"It's my neck. I can't move it. I think it's broken."

"Don't try to move." I examined his neck and could see nothing. I brought him a cup of tea and a morphine pill. When the pain lessened I went downstairs and called the Princess Margaret Hospital.

"Bring him in now. I'll admit him," Dr. Catton, who was newly assigned to Victor's case, urged. "We'll X-ray him right away."

I called the Canadian Cancer Society and was told all the volunteer drivers had left for the day.

"I'll be able to go on the bus," Victor said. He was dressed and more mobile now that the morphine was working, although the pain was still bad.

We were at the hospital a few hours later where he was taken immediately for X-rays.

"Mr. Newton, you have a small fracture in the upper vertebrae of your neck. This is the result of metastatic disease from the prostate cancer weakening your bones. You will have to stay in the hospital for at least a week while we radiate the area. The radiation should help heal the fracture and alleviate the pain. In the meantime, we will give you morphine intravenously." Dr. Catton turned to go. "I'll see you in the morning."

One week after his release from the hospital he was back again. This time it was his spine. I could hardly get him dressed because of the excruciating pain he felt with the least movement. Again I called Dr. Catton and again he wanted him admitted immediately.

"The bus is out of the question," I told my neighbour Mary, "and the Cancer Society only has room left for one passenger in their volunteer driver's program. All seats are taken. Victor won't go without me."

"Why don't you hire a limousine," she suggested.

"What a wonderful idea. I can put a pillow and blanket in the car."

Before long we were on our way to Toronto in a white stretch limousine and within two hours we were helped into the Princess Margaret Hospital where Victor received the last radiation to his spine. One of the doctors called it "palliative radiation," meaning that it was meant to relieve the pain and treat the disease without hope of curing it. Again we were told he would be in the hospital at least a week.

I stayed at an old hotel close to the hospital. I usually arrived on Victor's floor at 9:00 a.m. and stayed with him until nine at night, taking care of his needs and watching like a hawk to make sure he received his medication on time.

With the shortage of nursing staff in all hospitals things sometimes go wrong. On one occasion, he was supposed to be receiving morphine intravenously but he was still in terrible pain. When two hours had passed I went to the nurse's station and voiced my concern. Then, and a number of times later, I was told the morphine would kick in soon.

I finally demanded to see a doctor and the nurse checked the IV only to discover that it had not been turned on. From then on I watched to see how it was done.

Once Victor asked for a glycerine suppository to help him move his bowels. He did not get one. After two days, I purchased some at the drugstore for him. The morphine caused him to become incontinent at night which embarrassed him and the nurse fixed a plastic bag with tape around his penis to catch the urine that leaked while he was sleeping. I was horrified when I discovered that the nurse had torn the skin, along with the tape, from his penis. I went to the drugstore immediately and brought back an antibiotic ointment, cleaned the cut, and applied the healing salve.

"Victor dear, why didn't you say something?" I asked gently.

"I don't want to bother anybody. They're pretty busy," he said, almost like a child.

A week later I was thrilled to see that Victor was feeling

better. The good old radiation was working again. "Look what I bought for you," I said.

"Good grief. Christmas is three weeks away," he said. "What's this all about?"

"Oh, just a few things I thought you might like," I said. "Aren't you going to open it?"

Victor looked at the navy lambswool sweater and the soft blue checked shirt. I had always chosen colours he liked and I knew he would fuss and say I shouldn't spend the money, but he was pleased, too.

"I bought you these, too." I pulled a pair of pyjamas from the bag. We both laughed. The night before, Victor's new room-mate, an elderly priest who was suffering from brain cancer, came out of the bathroom wearing Victor's pyjamas. It was apparent that he was confused, and I took it upon myself to feed him when no one was available and to do little things that made a difference to him, like dialling a telephone number or cleaning his glasses.

One evening I heard him humming a familiar old hymn I recognized from my childhood and I sang it for him, along with a few more. He was thoroughly enjoying himself and asked me to sing a few Irish songs. Nurses and patients alike filed into the room to find out where the singing was coming from.

"That's my sweetheart," Victor said proudly.

"Not any longer, she's mine," Father O'Neil said, to everyone's surprise. The old priest died a few days later.

~

"Where's Victor?"

"Oh, he's not here," Victor's new roommate, Mario, said, coming out of the bathroom. I looked around the room.

"He said to tell you Room 202." Mario shuffled to the hall pointing me in the right direction.

"There he is," I said. I walked to Victor who was standing by a man in a wheelchair.

"Sweetheart, this is Bill Barker. Bill knows an old friend of mine, Don Shaw."

"How are you, Bill?" I asked, noticing Bill's yellow pallor.

"I'll be fine if I can just get these damn legs going." He pulled at one of his legs and raised it a few inches.

We learned that Bill, too, had prostate cancer metastasized to his spine. His legs had been paralyzed for a week but he was confident that radiation was going to restore him to full mobility. He was to receive treatment that afternoon.

"Now where is that woman?" Bill sounded agitated as he looked towards the elevator. "I'm waiting for my wife, Shirley," he explained. "Here she is now." Bill rolled his chair in the direction of the small blonde woman, calling "So long" over his shoulder to Victor and me.

The next morning, while passing his room, I peeked in to say hello. Bill was very upset. A tray of food was on the floor. Some bits of food still clung to the screen of the full-size television in his private room.

"Can I help?" I asked, knowing that Bill needed assistance to get out of bed.

"No thanks. That son-of-a-bitch came in here this morning and told me I'm not going to get better. I asked him if the feeling would come back in my legs and he just about said I was going to die." Bill had called his wife, Shirley, and she was on her way.

I was very careful with my words. "That doctor is an intern, Bill. Don't let him upset you. Wait and talk to your own doctor." I walked towards Victor who was standing in the doorway of his room, his brow furrowed. We could hear Bill yelling at the nurses.

"Bill is a millionaire contractor," he told me. "He lives in Rosedale." I was not impressed.

"Cancer is a great equalizer," I said thoughtfully.

Later that day we were given the grim news that the tumours growing in Victor's spine would compress his spinal cord and he too would become paralyzed, possibly in as little as three months. He was also told that he could go home.

He took the news bravely. While he packed his things, I checked with the doctor one last time before leaving the hospital.

"Mrs. Newton," Dr. Catton said, averting his eyes. "It would be best at this stage of your husband's disease if you do not bring him back. If he should need medical intervention – and he will, in a palliative form – then I think it would be best to have your family doctor in Peterborough look after him. You see, Mrs. Newton," the doctor continued, "if you bring him back again, we will just put him in the hospital and he will die here."

My throat tightened and my eyes filled with tears. I tried desperately not to cry. "Will you do one more thing for me, Doctor?" I asked.

"Of course, Mrs. Newton. What is it?" Dr. Catton had his hand on my arm.

"Will you give him one more appointment? I don't mean we will keep it. You see, the Princess Margaret Hospital has been his lifeline for ten years, his hope. I don't want to take his hope away."

"Certainly, Mrs. Newton. I'll make it out for six weeks from now. Call me if I can be of any help, any time." Dr. Catton walked away, his head lowered. He had just executed the hardest part of his duty as a physician. The part that he could not fix.

~

At home Victor's pain worsened and although he was under the best pain control possible – he was taking morphine three times daily – he still suffered immensely. He began to feel weakness in his legs more each day until he was no longer able to walk downstairs in the morning.

I turned the living room into a bedroom at night. Victor slept on the love-seat which had a pull-out bed and I slept on the chesterfield next to him. Each day he made a great effort to walk.

"Are you sure, Victor dear?" I asked, as I watched the pitiful struggle.

"I've got to," he replied, leaning more heavily on me each time. He insisted on trying to walk several times a day. I would walk with him from the living room through to the end of the dining room where he would pause and watch the children running back and forth to the variety store. Cars and trucks drove up and down the street, a dog barked, a door opened and closed, and the snow fell. The world was alive and moving but he no longer felt part of it. He wanted to. He had always had a powerful passion for life, but now he was filled with anxiety and uncertainty. What he wanted was reassurance. Although I kept his spirits up as much as I was able, he felt trapped in the nether world of cancer and all it contained.

≈

Dr. Leger handed me his coat and took three long strides across the room, extending his hand to Victor.

"Thank you for coming, Doctor." Victor stood up a little shakily.

"So how are you today?" inquired Dr. Leger. He reminded me of a young Gregory Peck as he pulled his stethoscope from his pocket and listened to Victor's chest.

"Well, I seem to be getting weaker in the legs each day." Victor kept his gaze on the doctor's angular face.

"Of course, you have prostate cancer all through you now," the doctor said, glancing from Victor to me.

The room fell silent. I sat close to Victor, my arm linked in his. "How long do I have?" Victor asked the question because he felt he had to. The doctor was expecting it.

"I don't know. Two weeks, a month, possibly two."

Victor turned white. "Oh, I can't listen to this," he said. He made an attempt to stand up. I was shocked.

The doctor stood up. "Increase the Dilaudid if you have more pain." He stopped and, looking at a painting, said, "I like that one. Call me if you need me, Mrs. Newton."

~

"Victor dear, how awful," I said, after the doctor had gone. "He doesn't know everything, only God knows." I looked at Victor's saddened face and I thought my heart would break. I felt such sorrow. I hated myself for not speaking up, but I also knew that Dr. Leger would be needed.

We were told when we chose him to be our family physician that he was an excellent doctor, dedicated and good at his craft, but he could also be blunt. What the doctor said and how he said it had a powerful effect on Victor.

"Don't blame him. I asked for it," Victor said, feeling fear turn to nausea in his stomach.

"Well, if you ask me he has a lot to learn about bedside manner." I cradled Victor and kissed his eyelids and forehead. He wept quietly. "I'm here, Vitts. I'm right here always."

~

It was Christmas Eve. I decorated a small tree while Victor sat on the chesterfield and watched.

"You're doing a great job, sweetheart. You always do." Suddenly, he was stricken with such pain and was in such obvious distress that I called for an ambulance. At the hospital he was found to have a blockage in the urethra and a small procedure was performed by the urologist to correct it. Victor was released and sent home by ambulance the following day, Christmas.

There wasn't any Christmas dinner. Everything seemed frivolous and unimportant. I got Victor settled for the night. I walked to the window. A light snow was falling, melting as it hit the pavement.

"Are you looking at your Christmas candy, sweetheart?" Victor asked, as he watched me standing quietly at the window.

"Yes I am, Vitts. You're reading my mind. The pavement is wet and the stoplights are reflected in it; yellow, red, and green, just like the Christmas candy." I turned at the sound of his sobs and went to him.

"I had a vision of you looking at your Christmas candy and someone had his arms around you but it wasn't me," he said tearfully.

"Victor darling, it will always be you. There could never be anyone else. I love only you and my love will never die."

∾

A few days later, my brother Joe arrived from Toronto. Joe was himself an oil artist and a great admirer of Victor's work. He was also a close friend. He had spent many hours talking to Victor about great artists. Victor would actually forget about his sickness and become animated while talking to Joe, but after a little while, his pain would remind him that nothing had changed.

He became very anxious when Joe had to leave, but Joe promised to return in one week and stay longer. Later, when Joe called me, he said, "I hadn't realized how very sick Victor is. I kept seeing him all the way home, trying to maintain his dignity, and yet I have the feeling he knows his story is coming to an end."

"He knows," I said.

As the tumours compressed Victor's spinal cord he felt the sensation of a thousand insects crawling inside his legs. I gave him the morphine but it did not relieve the crawling feeling, which was driving him crazy. Sometimes while sitting quietly watching television he would suddenly shriek and stamp his feet.

"Oh, I can't stand it," he moaned.

"Victor dear, what can we do?" I fell to my knees and massaged his legs, trying an assortment of remedies, hot towels, cold towels, Bengay, and Hot Ice. Nothing helped. I called Dr. Catton at the Princess Margaret Hospital.

"He is going to have this sensation until a total paralysis occurs, Mrs. Newton, and that should be soon, within days. I expect he will expire shortly after that, but I wouldn't underestimate him. Your husband is a very powerful individual," he added.

The nerve spasms worsened and Victor writhed in torment while I prayed for the paralysis to set in and give him some relief. A few days later the spasms were gone. I rented a wheelchair and a bedpan from a surgical supply house.

I was lifting Victor now from the wheelchair to the chesterfield and from the wheelchair to the bed. At first he was able to help me by using the strength in his upper body and arms to raise himself when I lifted him and together we would manage to get him onto the bedpan. But now his bowels were suffering paralysis and although he had the urge, he was unable to move them.

I was feeling the strain. Victor had lost what strength he had and I was alone with no one to help me lift him. One evening I knelt beside him and prayed to God, asking for strength. The next time I lifted him I did not feel his weight and told him so. "God answered my prayers," I said, covering him with the duvet.

∼

"Are you ready for home care?" Dr. Leger asked when I called to have Victor's prescription refilled.

"I could use some help," I replied.

That afternoon a home care case manager came to the house and was shocked to find I had been caring for Victor alone. She explained that I was not to worry about paying for their services because they were funded by O.H.I.P. "You will need a hospital bed and a Hoyer lift, a commode and surgical supplies, dressing pads, and so on," she said. "A nurse from the Victorian Order of Nurses will call in every day, possibly in the evening as well, and I am going to arrange for a Red Cross Homemaker to come in twice a week to give you a break, Mrs. Newton. You need rest."

When she had gone we felt as though a whirlwind had blown through the house, a welcoming, caring whirlwind.

∼

Victor watched for the mailman each day as though he were expecting a special letter, but, except for a few Christmas cards, there were no letters for him and no visitors over the holidays. I kept the family informed of his condition and appealed to them for much-needed financial help. We had not sold a painting for more than four months and the pension barely covered the mortgage and utilities. There was no money to fix the upstairs plumbing and I had to close off the bathroom entirely. "Thank God for the sink and toilet downstairs," I told Joe. Victor became upset whenever I suggested we ask his family for help. "I don't want to niggle at their comfort, especially at Christmas time," he said. I called his nephew Ronnie on the upstairs extension and asked him to approach the rest of the family for me. They all sent a few hundred dollars, some without a note. The money paid the back bills and I was grateful. I did not tell Victor about the call.

Finally Victor wrote to his brother Tom, asking him to appeal to the rest of the family to pay for his funeral. "Audrey just doesn't have the money," he wrote, as tears filled his eyes and his hand trembled. It was a poignant appeal, painfully written. He ended it with the words, "I love my brother Tom."

I called the girls and told them their father was in a wheelchair and that they should come and see him as soon as possible. They came the following Sunday and stayed a few hours.

I said, "Your dad has made his peace with God and has prepared his way."

Sandy went to the side of the wheelchair. "Well, just as long as you're not frightened," she said.

Laurie kept her place on the chesterfield. They kissed him goodbye and promised to call.

Joe returned. This time he could stay a week. Victor was delighted. "Good ole Joe," he said affectionately.

The hospital supplies were delivered, including the bed. For some reason Victor was not satisfied with the placement of the bed. No matter where I moved it he wasn't satisfied. He became increasingly agitated and near tears.

"Why don't we leave it here just for tonight, Vitts? You can try it out and if you don't like it we can always move it in the morning." I pushed the bed to the centre of the room. From there he could see anyone coming up onto the verandah through the front glass door. He could also see the television if he wished and I would sleep next to him on the chesterfield. The next day he had forgotten about the placement of the bed and it remained where it was.

To give him a change of position, an attempt was made to lift him out of bed with the Hoyer hydraulic lift. Victor screamed in pain. His spine was so fragile that any further attempt was out of the question, so he lay imprisoned in bed and body. Joe and I moved him from side to side and massaged his legs hourly. The pressure sores became larger, covering his entire tailbone. When he was turned on his side, a sore would quickly form on his hip. His bowels became paralyzed and had to be disimpacted by the nurse with her gloved finger. He also had a permanent catheter to carry away the urine, which I measured each morning before I bathed him and fed him his breakfast.

There seemed to be a lot of activity the first two weeks of his invalidism. The V.O.N. nurse came morning and night and the home care people busied themselves in the kitchen. Joe made tea for the nurses as they set up their supplies.

Victor was now considered to be under palliative complex care, which meant care to keep him comfortable and pain-free, but without hope of curing him. I prepared his meals. He was still eating a little each day, mostly soft but palatable foods, nothing he would have to chew because he no longer had the strength.

Whenever the telephone rang Victor became very alert and picked up the extension. He would not speak but he always listened so I was careful not to discuss his terminal state. When there were no calls, he became depressed.

Joe and a couple of friends who came to see Victor tried to comfort him but he would not be comforted. He began to cough uncontrollably, spitting up large amounts of blood. Everyone was quietly alarmed.

I called Dr. Leger, who explained that the large aorta could rupture and he would bleed from all openings. Dr. Leger asked me if I was prepared to take it or did I want to put Victor in the hospital.

"No, we'll carry on," I said. "I am not putting him in the hospital unless there is something they can do for him that can't be done at home."

A few dear friends called in to see Victor and to say goodbye. Peter, a big rugged Dutchman, had been one of his closest golf buddies. Victor was very glad to see him. They were shaking hands when, suddenly, Peter reached down and put his arms around Victor and kissed him. Victor tried to overcome his own feelings.

"That man kissed me," he said.

Joe chuckled. "That's okay, Victor. Peter was trying to tell you how much he loves you."

During the next few days Victor continued to cough up blood from his lungs. He was becoming weaker, but remained mentally alert. He still listened for the telephone to ring, as though he was expecting someone to call, but no calls came.

Finally his brother Tom telephoned and said to tell Victor not to worry about the burial expenses, that they would be taken care of. Victor had picked up the phone near his bed and quietly replaced the receiver. I saw the helpless look on his face and he averted his eyes when I sat next to his bed.

"Victor dear, I want you to know something." I took his hand. "I'll pay back every dollar that is loaned or given to us. I promise. You have no reason to lower your head, Victor." I reached over and raised his chin. "No one will take your dignity from you while I am here. I promise, sweetheart."

He looked at me through tear-filled eyes. "My fighter, I know you will, you proud Cape Bretoner. Thank you, sweetheart," he said, and he fell into a deep sleep.

∽

In the next few days Victor seemed determined to be his old self as much as possible. He took an interest in everything, what was on television, news, neighbours. He was making a valiant effort to regain a little control of his life, most of which had been taken over by the cancer, medical staff, and me. There was little left for him.

I gave him as much as possible. I gave him the remote control and placed a flashlight, pen, and paper on his bedside table. When his Timex watch stopped I went out and bought him a new one immediately. I gave him a choice of what he would like to eat and drink and when he would like the lights on or off, anything that would keep him interested and involved.

When the V.O.N. nurse, Ericka, was leaving one morning she asked if he wanted anything else and he said, "Yes, I want to see my wife's beautiful legs." Ericka blushed, surprised.

Later she told me, "I'm going through a divorce, Mrs. Newton. I hope I find a love like yours some day." She had tears in her eyes as she left the house.

Victor asked for his father's Bible. He had been reading the old Bible for years, after his diagnosis of cancer. I opened the book to the Psalms and read some of his favourite verses.

"Victor has a strong will to live," I told Joe. "He's no quitter."

"God love him. He won't see the tulips bloom," Joe said. "It's late February. Another two months before spring. He told me yesterday that he would like to see the garden one more time."

"Victor is going to see the tulips," I said. I dialled a local florist. "I want a hundred tulips, all colours, and I would like them now," I told the woman who answered the phone.

The tulips arrived, great bunches of them, in brilliant yellow, red, pink, and white. I arranged them in containers all around the room so that no matter where Victor looked he saw tulips.

"Beautiful," he said, his voice getting weaker. "Beautiful."

~

Over the next few days Victor struggled. His laboured breathing could be heard all through the house. I called the girls and told them that their father's condition had worsened rapidly, and they should come and see him as soon as possible.

Laurie was unable to come because of recent surgery. However, Sandy and her husband, Doug, arrived and stayed most of the following day, Sunday. Doug sat in the kitchen with Joe, and Sandy sat by her father's bed. Victor continued to cough up blood from his lungs every few minutes, closing his eyes, exhausted.

Sandy kissed her father and said goodbye. On her way out she looked back and bit her lip. Victor raised his hand and waved goodbye.

"What time it is?" he whispered. "I don't like the nights."

"It's eleven o'clock, but it will be morning before you know it, Vitts." I held his hand and Joe held the other one. He looked at Joe.

"I want you to know that you are my dearest and best friend," he paused, "but I love Audrey more," he added.

Joe put his hand on Victor's shoulder. Overcome with emotion, he left the room.

All through the night Victor struggled to breathe. He could no longer cough or spit and he weakened rapidly as he fell in and out of an exhausted sleep. I had the bed in a sitting position to help him breathe.

At eight in the morning he opened his eyes again. I was leaning over him wiping his mouth. With his last ounce of strength he raised his head and kissed me on the cheek.

"Victor dear, it's morning. It's a beautiful sunny morning," I said.

But Victor did not hear me. He had reached the top of the mountain. *What do I do now?* he wondered as he looked around. *Which way do I go?* He tried to remember what Audrey had said about the mountain. Positioning his skis on the edge, he took one last breath and pushed off towards the light.

~

Victor died on February 24, 1992, at 8:10 a.m. He is resting at the site we chose in Little Lake Cemetery in Peterborough. I often visit the site. In my own way, I continue to share my life with Vitts.

Victor's brother Chuck passed away on November 6, 1993, after a three-year battle with urinary-related cancer. His golf buddy, Peter, was diagnosed in May 1993 with prostate cancer.

While writing this book, I became aware of more than a dozen people who are dealing with family members suffering from prostate cancer. Early detection is the only way to stop this disease. If a man in your life is over forty, urge him to make an appointment for a check-up by his doctor now. He should tell his friends to do the same.

The Way Ahead

New Developments

Things are changing in the treatment of prostate cancer just
as they are in virtually all other areas of medicine. New drugs
have been introduced since Victor's prostate cancer was diagnosed in 1981. New hormone therapy drugs are available with
fewer side effects. New surgical techniques have been developed. Radical prostatectomy is no longer the dangerous operation it once was. The estimated hospital stay for men who have
undergone the procedure is now about a week to ten days,
depending upon the patient's age and the state of his health.
The recovery period, however, could be as long as six months.
Dr. Patrick C. Walsh at the Johns Hopkins University Hospital,
Baltimore, Maryland, has come up with a new surgical tech-
nique used in radical prostatectomy that spares the nerve
bundles that contribute to sexual function. Again, recovery of
potency depends upon the age and state of health of the patient
and could take anywhere from six months to a year. These new

discoveries have greatly improved the quality and length of life of the prostate cancer sufferer.

Public awareness of prostate cancer has increased dramatically in recent years. Prostate cancer support groups are being formed all over Canada and the United States. Partly because more men are living longer, more men are also contracting prostate cancer. Its prevalence is finally being recognized. Prominent, high-profile men are revealing their cases to the media. The U.S. senator and presidential candidate Robert Dole and General Norman Schwarzkopf, hero of the Gulf War, are two among many men who are speaking openly about their prostate cancer. Roger Moore, Karl Malden, Sydney Poitier, Jerry Lewis, and Robert Goulet are all prostate cancer survivors. Floyd Laughren, former Ontario finance minister, recently underwent surgery for prostate cancer and is confident of a cure. So this is the good news. If detected early enough, prostate cancer is curable. Even when the cancer is found in the lymphatic system, like Victor's, the possibility of living a long, productive life is real.

I'm on the committee of the Prostate Cancer Support Group in my city, and I know men who have survived for ten, fifteen, and even twenty years after their prostate cancer was diagnosed.

Some Prostate Cancer Statistics

Since the 1960s, the number of prostate cancer cases has risen dramatically. Fourteen thousand new cases are expected in Canada this year, of which 4,000 will prove fatal. In the United States, the figures are of course much higher – 200,000 new cases and approximately 40,000 deaths. Prostate cancer is the second leading cause of all cancer deaths in men, following closely behind lung cancer.

The incidence of prostate cancer in white males is 88 in 100,000, as compared to 132 in 100,000 African Americans. The rate for Asian men is much lower, with only 4 in 100,000; however, when they immigrate to North America, the rate climbs rapidly.

Researchers are looking at high-fat diets in relation to all cancers, including prostate cancer. Environmental factors are also being closely studied.

The last decade will go down in medical history as the decade of prostate cancer enlightenment. The disease is no longer the silent killer it once was. Men are speaking more openly and comfortably about their prostates. The next decade will prove to be even more challenging, as researchers seek out more sophisticated tests to identify and destroy early prostate cancers. Awareness of prostate cancer will also help generate the much-needed funding for the all-important research and study of prostate cancer. It has been reported that prostate cancer cells can be found in one-third of men over the age of fifty. However, the median age of diagnosis is seventy-one years.

There is one positive thing that can be said about prostate cancer – it is a slow-growing disease. Most men die with it, rather than of it. Nevertheless, the fight for earlier diagnosis, better treatment, and an ultimate cure, continues.

A few months after Victor's death in 1992, I received separate phone calls from two of his golfing buddies. They were concerned because they, too, had been making extra trips to the bathroom at night. One of them said that he knew Victor and I had been comfortable talking about his prostate cancer so he, in turn, was comfortable asking me about it. It was this conversation that led me to the realization that there is a need for accurate information on the subject written in a way that both men and women can easily understand.

Many people assisted me in attempting to meet this need. A number of doctors generously took the time to read the manuscript at different stages and advised me on the accuracy of the medical information. Their assistance, of course, does not mean that they agree in all respects with the manner in which the material is presented. My sincere thanks to: Dr. Robert P. Myers, Consultant at the Mayo Clinic, and Professor of Urology at the Mayo Graduate School of Medicine in Rochester, Minnesota; Dr. Charles N. Catton, radiation oncologist at the Princess Margaret Hospital, Toronto, and Assistant

Professor at the University of Toronto; Dr. E.J. Hambley and Dr. F.C. Meade, urologists in the city of Peterborough, Ontario.

Thanks to Doug Cruthers and his daughter Laurie Coulter for guiding me in the right direction.

My thanks to my editor, Jonathan Webb, for bravely taking on a first-time author, and to my publisher, McClelland & Stewart.

I am especially indebted to my brother, Joe-Allen Currie, whose love and faith in my ability to write this book spurred me on.

Special thanks to Susan Howson in the beginning, Valerie Lewis in the middle, and Cindy MacFarlane all the way.

Thanks to my son, Robert, who first typed my manuscript into his computer and presented me with the disk.

Finally, my thanks to the many prostate cancer survivors I met along the way who shared their stories and deep feelings of hope and fear with me. I will always be here for you.

Organizations

American Cancer Society (ACS)
The American Cancer Society provides general information, free publications on topics of interest to cancer patients and their supporters, and information about support groups. Phone numbers of regional offices are listed in the telephone directory, or call their 1-800 number.

American Cancer Society information line:
1-800-227-2345

Canadian Cancer Society (CCS)
There are branches of the Canadian Cancer Society across the country. They are an invaluable source of information, guidance and support. Among other resources offered are free booklets on prostate cancer, available in both French and English, including the following titles: *Facts on Prostate Cancer; Prostate Cancer; Radiation Therapy and You: A Guide for Self-Help during Treatment; Pain Relief: Information for People with Cancer and Their Families.*

Canadian Cancer Society Provincial Offices:

Alberta / Northwest Territories
Suite 200, 2424 – 4th Street S.W.
Calgary, Alberta T2S 2T4
(403) 228-4487

British Columbia and Yukon
565 W. 10th Avenue
Vancouver, British Columbia V5Z 4J4
(604) 872-4400

Manitoba
193 Sherbrooke Street
Winnipeg, Manitoba R3C 2B7
(204) 774-7483

New Brunswick
133 Prince William Street
Saint John, New Brunswick E2L 3T5
(506) 634-6272

Newfoundland and Labrador
P.O. Box 8921, Chimo Building
St. John's, Newfoundland A1B 3R9
(709) 753-6520

Nova Scotia
Suite 1, 5826 South Street
Halifax, Nova Scotia B3H 1S6
(902) 423-6183

Ontario
1639 Yonge Street
Toronto, Ontario M4T 2W6
(416) 488-5400

Prince Edward Island
131 Water Street, 2nd floor
Charlottetown, P.E.I. C1A 7K2
(902) 566-4007

Quebec
5151 boul. L'Assomption
Montreal, Quebec H1T 4A9
(514) 255-5151

Saskatchewan
Suite 201, 2445 – 13th Avenue
Regina, Saskatchewan S4P 0W1
(306) 757-4260

In addition to the provincial offices, the Canadian Cancer Society currently sponsors three Cancer Information Service Lines:

British Columbia / Yukon
In Vancouver: (604) 879-2323
Outside Vancouver: 1-800-663-4242
Fax: (604) 879-9267

Ontario
In Toronto/Hamilton: (905) 387-1153
Outside Toronto/Hamilton: 1-800-263-6750
Fax: (905) 387-0376

Quebec
In Montreal: (514) 522-6237
Outside Montreal: 1-800-361-4212

Support Groups

There are many support groups for people living with prostate cancer. Some are affiliated with the Canadian Cancer Society; some are organized by hospitals; others are community based. To contact the support group nearest you, call the Canadian Cancer Society office nearest you or ask your doctor.

US TOO Prostate Cancer Support Group

After undergoing a radical prostatectomy in 1989, Ed Kaps wanted to talk about it with someone, but he didn't know another man with prostate cancer. He decided to organize a support group for men with the disease and their families. During that first year Ed received more than ten thousand calls and letters from people wanting information on the disease. Today, US TOO support groups are being formed all over Canada and the United States. The groups are made up of people from all walks of life. They usually meet once a month. A guest speaker may be invited to give a talk on impotence, incontinence, nutrition and a variety of other subjects that may concern the prostate cancer survivor. Most men who attend these meetings find that they can tell their stories and reveal their feelings easily because they all share a common experience with the disease. This, in itself, can be a relief. The information made available through these meetings is invariably useful.

Man-to-Man

This group provides helpful information and education to men and their families about prostate cancer. For more information about this group, contact the Canadian Cancer Society, Central Toronto Unit, Suite 101, 20 Holly Street, Toronto.

Books

There are a great many books available about cancer and cancer treatments. More are being published all the time. The following titles are recommended as a place to begin your researches. Do, however, make use of your bookstore, public library and friends to find other sources of information.

Dollinger, Malin, M.D., Ernest H. Rosenbaum, M.D., and Greg Cable. *Everyone's Guide to Cancer Therapy: How Cancer is Diagnosed, Treated and Managed, Day to Day*. Toronto: Somerville House Publishing, 1992.

Goldenberg, S. Larry, M.D., *The Intelligent Patient Guide to Prostate Cancer*. Vancouver: Intelligent Patient Guide, 1992.

Morra, Marian, and Eve Potts. *Choices: Realistic Alternatives in Cancer Treatment*. New York: Avon, 1987.

The Merck Manual of Diagnosis and Therapy, which is mentioned in the text, is a clinical source used by doctors and pharmacists. Most people will find it of little use.